MW00526452

A Doctors Guide to
LIVING LONGER
AND BETTER

How to Thrive Throughout Your Retired Years...

Instead of Simply Surviving.

By Dr. Andrew Scanameo

Disclaimer

Regarding Expectations of Results – Dr. Andrew Scanameo and the publisher accept no liability for the use or misuse of the information contained in this book. There is no possibility of substantiating any claimed results made or supplying any objective evidence, whether financial, business related, spiritual or otherwise. Dr. Andrew Scanameo and the publisher strongly advise that you seek professional advice as appropriate before making any health decision. It can be assumed that no results are to be expected as a result of one's purchase of this book. Dr. Andrew Scanameo and the publisher do not and cannot make any representations, promises or guarantees of the effectiveness of this book. That being said, Dr. Andrew Scanameo and his associates, partners and affiliates firmly believe in the effectiveness of the methods put forth in this book.

Published by Inspired Solutions Publishing.

Las Vegas NV 89121 USA

CONTENTS

INTRODUCTION

Why I am writing this book...and why it is important.

What does "age" mean? Is age really, as the ever-optimistic saying goes, truly "nothing but a number"? From what each of us knows, from what each of us has seen in the lives of others, and possibly even in our own life, we know that this is not entirely accurate, right? We know that age is more than just a number; instead, age is a measurement of how long we have been on this Earth...and, as most of us have seen or experienced, how long we have been on this Earth will dictate everything from our mental health to our physical health to our level of expectancy for an enjoyable life.

As we get older, life gets harder...right? As we get older, possibilities begin to evaporate, and in the place of possibilities, many of us are faced with a none-too-pleasant reality. We spend most of our time shuttling back and forth between our home and the hospital. We have nurses visiting us at our bedside and injecting fluids into our body. The idea of "travel" becomes laughable; the idea of "an enjoyable retirement" seems like little more than a fairy tale. The ideas of "enjoying life" and, more than anything, "thinking about the future" may as well be the punch line to a depressing joke. "The future?" Many of us think when we hear others talk about their plans for those down-the-road years, "Yeah right, I'm just trying to survive in the present."

But what if this did not have to be the case?

What if there were more available to us in our post-work years?

What if it were possible for us to do more than simply "survive" into our 60s, 70s, 80s, and 90s? (Yes, you read that right, I did say 90s.) What if, instead, it was possible for us to *thrive*, for us to lead a full, enjoyable, rewarding life, and for us to truly feel fulfilled, deep into our "older years"? What if it were possible for life to be enjoyed, rather than for us to simply last through the years?

What if it were possible to *LIVE LONGER AND BETTER?*

Years ago, I decided that I wanted to find a new way in which to push myself physically. I wanted to find a new goal I could set for myself, a new accomplishment towards which I could build. I have always been a fairly active person. I was a lacrosse player, I spent three years in the United States Air Force, I have continued to work out regularly, and even now, in my 50s, I would rather play sports than watch them, but I wanted to have a "goal" towards which I could be working; a "long-term task" that would require me to work hard in order to accomplish it. I decided, after thinking about it, that I wanted to run a triathlon.

For months, I built toward this goal. I added to my workout regimen; I tailored this regimen specifically to ensure I would be able to accomplish this goal; I put in lots of time and hard work in order to reach a point where I felt comfortable that I would be able to compete in and (most importantly at the time) complete the triathlon I had set out to conquer.

The morning of the triathlon arrived at last, and I got up bright and early, ready to prove to myself and to the world that I could do this. Little did I know when I woke up that morning, however, that "finishing my first triathlon" would not be the experience that would stick with me the most on that day. Not by a long shot...

That morning, I met a man who changed my thinking forever. We did not spend much time together. We did not become friends or exchange contact information or even, for that matter, ever see each other again. But meeting that man altered my perspective forever. Meeting that man led me, when it comes down to it, to the place where I am today, living life the way I live it, and writing this book in order to help others do the same.

The man was 94 years old. And he was there that morning for the same reason I was there - to run a triathlon.

Maybe he finished second-to-last that morning. Maybe he did not clock his best time. But there he was anyway, 94 years old, running a triathlon.

What if this is what our post-work years are supposed to look like? What if retirement is about more than just sitting around and waiting for the time to pass, what if the ages of 60, 70, 80, and 90 are about more than just "surviving"? What if, instead, we are supposed to be able to use these years to enjoy life, live life to the fullest, and genuinely *thrive?*

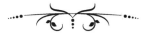

Even before I met that 94-year-old man running the triathlon, I was working in geriatric medicine, spending most of my time around patients in their 70s, 80s, and 90s, and with a practice based in Tallahassee, Florida, I have certainly had no shortage of patients and experiences with people in their "older years."

Even before I met that 94-year-old triathlete, I felt that I was far more progressive than most other doctors in my area of medicine. I was far more interested in helping individuals truly improve and truly "lead a better life," instead of simply helping them "feel more comfortable" as they deteriorated. But meeting that man helped to open my perspective even further. I realized just how full our lives have the capacity to be, no matter what age we are.

As we get deeper into this book, we will look more closely at my idea of the "exceptional retired individual," compared to the "conventional retired individual." But one of the major obstacles that stands between most older people and their opportunity to become an "exceptional retired individual" is, quite simply, their concept of what the ages of 60, 70, 80, and 90 look like.

Because they imagine these years are supposed to be "years of decline," and because the doctors they are visiting have no interest in dispelling this notion, they buy into this lie. They lead a lifestyle that perpetuates decline. And they fail to take hold of the bright future and the full life that is there for the taking. Instead of finding ways to continually improve their present and expand their future, they allow themselves to crumble physically and mentally; they allow doctors to overmedicate them; they slowly fade into nonexistence...even before they actually pass away.

For years, my practice has been focused on reversing this trend. Each and every day, I meet with people in their "older years" and aim to find ways in which I can help them lead better lives. I help them *improve* physically and mentally, instead of simply easing the downward trajectory. I help them move toward a brighter future, and I help them understand just how full life can still be, even at the place in life where they find themselves at the moment.

Put simply: each and every day, I strive to help patients *LIVE LONGER AND BETTER*. And the results I see from patients who buy into the belief that this is possible, the results I see from patients who are willing to do what they must do in order to "thrive" instead of simply "survive," are astonishing. The health of patients begins to improve; their lives begin to become more full, and their futures begin to become brighter. I see it every day.

But I have come to realize that there is only so much I can do. As I continue to practice at my clinic each day and see patients on a case-by-case basis, I fail to reach the hundreds of millions of people in their 60s, 70s, 80s, and 90s who live in other parts of the world... and I fail to reach the hundreds of millions of people in their 40s and 50s who could actually be taking steps in their own "present" to ensure that they have a healthy, fulfilling future. It was the recognition of these limitations that led me to the idea of writing this book.

Before we get any deeper into this book, you need to realize that the title of this book is not a marketing ploy. The point behind this book is not, "Yes, some of you can *LIVE LONGER AND BETTER*, but most of you will still be left simply easing your decline." No.

The title of this book is, truly, the goal we are driving toward, and it is something I firmly believe: each and every one of us has the ability to LIVE LONGER AND BETTER.

You have the ability to *LIVE LONGER AND BETTER.*

Once you grasp this, once you begin to believe that this is true, and once you decide that this is something you truly want for yourself, you will be in a position to chase this future (yes, "future," no matter how old you are.). You will be ready to put yourself in the position to *LIVE LONGER AND BETTER.*

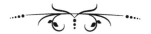

I'll be honest with you: I am expecting that you will read this entire book. After all, it is not too terribly long, and it is absolutely packed with valuable knowledge and information that will help you to *LIVE LONGER AND BETTER.* Throughout this book, I will essentially be leading you step-by-step toward the path you must follow in order to see the reality of this idea in your own life.

So, how about it? Can we agree that you will invest the few hours required of you in order to read this book in its entirety? Okay, good. Before we get started with the meat of this book, then, I want to give you an idea of exactly what this book is going to look like, and what this book will cover.

One of the things I see far too often from patients who come to me after they have seen other doctors is that they visit my office with a concept that there is nothing for them to do at this point in their life but wait around for death in as comfortable a manner as possible. Of course, no patients come right out and say things quite so blatantly, but this is the foundation on which their mindset is built. And you know why they feel this way? Beyond the fact that they have seen this "truth" in the lives of those around them, this "truth" has also been encouraged by doctors.

I see patients who are on medication that is causing health complications...but because this medicine does a bit to ease pain or discomfort, other doctors keep this medicine going. I see patients who come to me because they are looking to have their discomfort removed... patients who have no concept of the alternate reality available to them.

I see patients who are ready to simply check out and fade away into nonexistence. I see patients who spend most of their day on the couch, and who do nothing active. I see patients who do nothing to keep their mind sharp, and who have no concept of monitoring their emotional health and their spirituality. I see patients who are perfectly comfortable with the idea that this is what life is supposed to look like.

I also, however, see patients who latch onto the ideas I preach, patients who start taking whole-self steps, looking to improve their body, their mind, their emotions, and their spirituality, and who see marked improvements as a result. I see patients whose lives turn around when they start living *intentionally*. I see patients who begin to *thrive*. And this is the purpose of this book.

After reading this book, you will understand the manner in which your body, your mind, your emotions, and your spirituality tie together. And more importantly, you will understand what you should be doing in order to improve all these areas of your life.

As you read this book, then, I encourage you to do so with an open mind. I write this book realizing that some of the things I say in here may not necessarily line up with the things you have heard from other doctors, and as such, I want to implore you to ask yourself, "What are the results that I am seeing from what these other doctors are saying?" Are you seeing improvements in your own life (or in the lives of others) by following the conventional medical approaches to progressing through the later years of life?

Each of us has more say over the state of our body than conventional medicine gives us credit for, and in order to reach a point where you are living life to the fullest, in order to reach a place from which you are *LIVING LONGER AND BETTER*, you need to be willing to shun some of the conventional thinking.

If you are willing to read this book with an open mind, this book has the capacity to change your life. This book has the ability to help you "thrive" through your older years, to help you become, in short, an "exceptional retired individual." This book has the ability to help you *LIVE LONGER AND BETTER*. And if you are willing to read this book with an open mind and listen to the things it says, this is exactly what your future (yes, future) will look like.

As you read this book, pay attention to the thoughts in it that you have perhaps failed to think about yourself. Look for the ways in which you can incorporate into your own life the principles presented in this book. Determine what you can (and should) be doing differently in order to reach the goal of *LIVING LONGER AND BETTER.*

And then, when you finish reading this book, tell others about it. Let them know that there is more to life, more to "old age," than what most have trapped themselves into imagining. Let them know that it is possible for them to thrive, that it is possible for them to be an "exceptional retired individual." Let them know that they can *LIVE LONGER AND BETTER.*

Get the message out there. Together, we can change the way we see old age. Together, we can change the world.

WHAT IT MEANS TO
LIVE BETTER

It is not enough to simply "survive." It is time to start thriving.

"Working toward retirement." It's a phrase we hear all too frequently, a phrase that implies that the purpose of the years between the ages of 20 and 60 is to set ourselves up for those wonderful, post-work years of retirement. This phrase indicates a perceived idea that those years after the age of 60 will be something of a "golden era" in our lives; that we will retire and (finally) be able to do what we want to do…that we will be able to truly enjoy life at last.

"Wait," you may be saying right now, "who are you talking to?" You may be wondering if I am speaking to individuals who are already retired (Well, that's the audience this book is intended for, isn't it?), or if I am instead speaking to individuals who are still in those "ages 20 to 60" years.

The answer? I am speaking to both.

One of the core ideas behind this book is to help retired individuals reach a place from which they will be able to truly live life, a place from which such individuals will be able to THRIVE, instead of simply surviving.

But while this book certainly aims to help retired individuals to turn the corner and start "really living" at last, I also know that many of you reading this are doing so because you want to find out how you can help your parents or grandparents to "live longer and better." One thing to realize, however, is that it is always best to start on this path *NOW*, regardless of what "now" is to you at the moment.

The principles behind this idea are similar to the principles of investing. While it is worth anyone's time, effort, and energy to invest their money and use it to build more money, there is a principle in investing called "Time value of money." This principle, essentially, brings to light the simple truth that the sooner you get started investing, the greater the long-term rewards will be. (No, I know, this is not a book about investing. But bear with me for just one second; this is going somewhere important, I promise.)

In sticking with our example of investing: let's take someone who has $1,000 to invest, and let's assume that this person is able to gain a standard return of 10% per year. If this person began investing this money at the age of 50, they would grow this money to $2,593 by the time they reach the age of 60. That's great, right?

But what if they started investing at the age of 40? By starting 10 years earlier, they would be able to turn that same $1,000 into $6,727 by the age of 60. And of course, we could go back even further and pretend this lucky individual began investing their $1,000 at the age of 20. In this instance, by the age of 60, they would have grown their original investment into $45,259. In other words, by investing their money four times longer, they would actually increase their profit by almost 30 times.

I bring all this up because I feel that the idea of "thriving" instead of "surviving," the idea of *LIVING BETTER*, becomes that much more powerful when we start on this path at the youngest possible age. If you are reading this book as a 60-year-old (or a 70-year-old, or an 80-year-old.), you can apply the principles within this book to your life, and you will be able to immediately see an improvement in your quality of life, will be able to apply these principles, that is, and immediately begin down the path of *LIVING BETTER*.

But if you are reading this as someone who is younger, it gets even better. You may have picked up this book because you wanted to figure out the ways in which you could help your parents or grandparents *LIVE LONGER AND BETTER* (or, heck, you may have picked up this book because your parents or grandparents themselves recommended it to you), but now that you are reading this book, it is time to realize that much of the information contained within these pages applies to you as well; at the place in your life where you are right now.

By beginning to live better at this very moment, the benefits will grow to an even greater extent in exactly the same way that $1,000 grew to an exponentially greater extent for the person who invested it for longer. The sooner you start investing into your own life, the greater the rewards you will reap over time.

Far too many people use their pre-retirement years to "work toward retirement," always imagining that things will magically become more wonderful in their life as soon as they reach the "Holy Grail" of those retirement years. These people fail to appreciate the journey, and along the way, they also fail to practice enjoying life. They fail, quite simply, to live better.

They say that practice makes perfect, right? Well, I'm here to tell you that this is absolutely true, and if you fail to practice *LIVING BETTER* in the years before you reach retirement, you will continue in this failure when retirement is finally upon you. Like so many others, you will end up leading a retired life in which the days bleed together, and in which you "hang around" as life passes you by...a life in which you fail to ever really get the most out of the precious time you have. I see it all the time, and it's time for this to stop. It's time for us to put an end to living mediocre lives. It's time for all of us to realize that it is possible for us to live better.

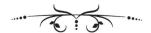

Let's take you on a vacation. That sounds nice, doesn't it? How about a beach vacation, I'm thinking the Bahamas. Sound good?

You fly into Nassau. It's a small airport, but it is clean and colorful. The people working at the airport are all smiling at you, they're all happy, all in love with life. When you walk outside, the air is warm, pleasant, not too hot, but just hot enough to let you know you are on vacation, and to let you know that some time on the beach is shortly in order.

You are staying on Paradise Island, just off the coast of New Providence, and you catch a taxi for the 20-minute ride to your resort. The cab driver is friendly and accommodating, very proud of his country, and of the beauty it offers. He points out landmarks to you as you cruise through the lush, green countryside, and as you then pass through the hustle and bustle of downtown Nassau.

Upon arriving at the resort, you head up to the room. You are on the 18th floor with a balcony and a breathtaking view of the calm, Caribbean waters stretching to eternity. After a swim in the ocean and a delicious dinner of local cuisine (try the conch salad; I know, it sounds a bit adventurous, but it's a local specialty, and you really cannot beat it), it's time to turn in for the night. You leave the door to the balcony open and fall asleep to the sounds of the ocean far below.

On your first full day of vacation, you have an excursion planned to Rose Island, a private island with a private beach and a quiet restaurant/bar overlooking the ocean. You take a boat to Rose Island with around 20 other people; the group of people on the boat will be the only people on Rose Island that day. It's a wonderful day, quiet, relaxing, and refreshing. You leave Rose Island at the end of the day feeling entirely replenished. You turn in early that night, once more falling asleep to the sounds of the ocean far below.

Day two of vacation, you have a horseback riding expedition planned. You have to wake up earlier than you really want to on vacation, but as you cruise through the countryside in the back of the taxi with the window down and the clear air streaming in through the window, you wake up entirely and begin to get excited about this opportunity to go horseback riding on the beach.

The waters on this side of the island are absolutely motionless, totally clear, see-through, and tranquil. You can see the colorful fish swimming several feet below the surface as your horse takes you along a leisurely stroll through the sand, and in front of you, your guide (whose personality is about as colorful as the fish beneath the surface of the water) tells you stories of the famous people he has led along this same path, on these same horses: Nicolas Cage, Sean Connery, Julia Roberts, and many, many more. It's a breathtaking experience, and it is far more fun than you even imagined it would be.

After another delicious dinner and another calm, relaxing night of sleep, you decide to use the third and final day of vacation to simply relax on the beach, to lounge in a lounge chair with a cold drink and your favorite book, and to soak up the sun and the quiet sound of the calm, Caribbean waters washing back and forth over the perfect white sand. At night, you sit on the balcony and watch the sun set over the water, and then you fall asleep with the door open with the sounds of the ocean rocking you to sleep once more...

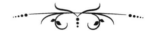

You're back home from vacation, back to the real world...back to life. For the first couple days, all you want to do is return to the Bahamas, return to that paradise in which you felt so tremendously relaxed, refreshed, and replenished. When the alarm clock goes off that first morning, when you roll out of bed and your feet hit the cold floor, and you shower to try to wake up and psyche yourself up for the day, all you can think about is how you wish you were still in the Bahamas, still enjoying vacation.

Someone cuts you off on the highway and nearly makes you spill your coffee. Traffic builds up, and you're stop-and-go for a while. Finally, you arrive at your office, and your "to do" stack has grown twice as much as you expected it to grow in your short time away. The morning drags on, and you find yourself glancing at your watch about once every three minutes. You begin to wonder if your watch is broken...you begin to wonder if time itself is broken. The morning seems to drag on for weeks.

You eat a cold sandwich for lunch and have a meeting in the afternoon that leaves you with even more work to catch up on. Finally, it's time to leave for home, and as you sit in traffic again. You decide you are going to plan another trip to the Bahamas. You are going to save up money and return to paradise again...

The next twelve months drag on just like this. There are a few highlights, but for the most part, your life consists of putting in your time at work so you can save up money and save up vacation days and return to the Bahamas for a few more wonderful days of vacation. You don't think about each day too much, beyond simply thinking about getting through that day. After all, it's just a work day, what is there to think about, really? What is there to enjoy? You put in your time with these work days so you can reach that vacation once more, and finally, after a full year has passed, you reach that vacation at last. You hop on a plane and fly to Nassau, and, for a few precious days, life is finally good...

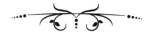

Do you see it? Do you see what we discovered in that little journey we just took? Do you see the similarities between that example and the way most people live life? When you think about it, it's sad. When you think about it, in fact, it's downright scary...

Life. We get one shot at it, right? We get one chance to walk through this journey, and yet, so many of us skip huge parts of the journey as we "look forward to the things toward which we are working." In some cases, those "things toward which we are working" are vacations we are planning or holidays we are looking forward to (holidays that, like a vacation, will give us a precious day or two away from work). In other cases, those "things toward which we are working" are the dreams of retirement, those dreams of the days when we will no longer have to work, and will have freedom at last.

And then, we retire, and what do we do? For many people, the first few weeks of retirement are great. There is so much extra time available. There is so much to catch up on, so much to enjoy, so much to do. It's like a long vacation. But then, the novelty wears off. We lose the enthusiasm for "doing nothing."

We find ourselves waking up, taking a quick shower (or sometimes not), then shuffling to our recliner and clicking on the television. We flip through channels, watching reruns of shows we used to like, watching morning shows, watching news reports. We watch a 30-minute segment in which a pair of super-tanned, enthusiastic individuals in their early-20s try to sell us the newest piece of "miracle workout equipment." We watch the entire 30-minute segment without even registering that this is what we are doing, without even registering that time is passing, and we are sitting in a recliner watching a 30-minute ad and otherwise doing absolutely nothing. That night, we turn in early. The next day, we do it all again...

For many people, this is what life becomes. The habit is formed during the "working years" of never really enjoying each day, but of instead "making it through each day" in order to reach one long-term goal or another (be it a vacation or that "long vacation" of retirement itself). And then, by the time we retire, we are so out of practice with enjoying life, so out of practice with getting the most out of life...so out of practice with *LIVING BETTER*, that we use retirement as a means to waste away. Life disappears like ice melting in the sun, leaving behind nothing at all.

It's sad.

It's scary.

But there is good news.

The good news? It's this:

There is a better way.

There is a life that is far greater, far more fulfilling, far more rewarding, than this.

The other good news? You can start this life at any point. Sure, as in our example with the individual investing $1,000, the younger you are when you begin the practice of *LIVING BETTER*, the more this "better life" will build on itself and create a truly enjoyable and rewarding existence. But even if you are 60 years old, or even if you are 70 years old, or even if you are 80 years old, there is a better way. There is an opportunity for life to become for you what life should be. There is a way for you to live better.

In order to illustrate what life can look like at its fullest, I like to always start with those years in which many falsely believe that it is impossible for life to actually be full, those years during which "work" dominates the majority of our hours...those years between the ages of 20 and 60 when so many people are doing nothing more than "striving toward retirement."

Even if you are already retired, and are asking, "But Dr. Andrew, how can I start living better *now*, as a retired individual?" This chapter is still for you. Over the next couple pages, I am going to paint a picture for you of what I see that often-elusive "better life" is looking like for someone who is still in their working years.

Of course, if this is the stage of life in which you currently exist yourself, if you are in those "ages 20 to 60" years, and are working each day, this section applies to you directly. But even if you are past this stage of life, take the time to read this section. As with any area of learning, advanced knowledge must build upon the knowledge that came before it. For those of you who are fortunate enough to be starting at a young age along the path toward *LIVING BETTER*, you will be able to start learning from experience and practice, and will reach those retirement years with a firm, first-hand grasp of exactly what it means to live life to the fullest.

But if you are already in those retirement years and, like so many others in the same boat as you, are wanting to learn what you can do differently to truly get the most out of life, one important step along the path will be understanding what "living better" looks like even before retirement is reached. The knowledge you need in order to enjoy life NOW will build upon the knowledge set forth in the next few paragraphs.

This is an illustration of what life could (and should) look like for someone still in those working years... someone wanting to live better starting now, instead of forever waiting until later.

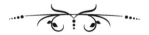

That vacation we took you on earlier sounded nice, didn't it? If you're like me, in fact, that section of this book made you wish you could pack your bags, hop on a plane, and enjoy those few days described in that section right now. (Heck, that section made me feel that way, and I wrote it myself.) But I want to take you on another journey right now...a journey that has nothing to do with "vacations."

I want to take you, instead, through a journey of a typical work day. I want to show you an alternative illustration, that is, of what a "typical work day" could (and should) look like. I want to paint a picture of a work day for someone who is *LIVING BETTER*, even as they go through what others may see as the mundane portions of life.

Once more, we are going to put you in the driver's seat for this journey. This is your "perfect work day" as you strive to "thrive," instead of living a life in which you simply survive...

You wake up to your alarm clock and do not even realize that you are already smiling. Another day is upon you. You swing your feet onto the cold floor and hurry to the shower, and you wake up more fully as the water washes over you. You step out of the shower and get dressed feeling refreshed, replenished, ready to go.

You sit down for a pleasant, relaxing breakfast and open that morning's newspaper. The steam from your mug of coffee seems to awaken your senses. When breakfast is finished, you step out into a crisp morning and stand on the front porch for a moment or two, simply breathing in the clean air before walking to your car and starting the long commute to work, one of your favorite parts of the day, as you are able to use this time to listen to the new audiobook you are making your way through (or are able to use this time to start learning a new language with those CDs you bought and have been meaning to finally get started on).

Someone cuts you off in traffic, and you chuckle. You feel bad for someone starting out their day in such an apparently combative and foul mood. Traffic builds up, but you don't really mind; after all, this gives you more time in the car to enjoy the start of the day.

When you show up at work, you notice that your "to do" pile seems to have doubled in size overnight. You can't say you particularly "love" work, but hey, it sure beats not having a job. You organize the "to do" pile and get started. "Well," you think, "there's only so much I can do in a day. I'll take care of as much of this as I can today, then I'll get back to it tomorrow." Better to be busy at work than to have nothing to do anyway, right?

At lunch, you decide to go for a walk. This is a bit of a departure from the norm, as you have asked for, and received, permission from your boss to have a "working lunch," which enables you to eat while working and continue plugging away during your lunch break. Most days, then, you leave work an hour early, and are able to use this extra time for a quality workout and for more time with your family.

On this day, however, the fresh air calls you, so you get your sandwich out of the way quickly, pull on your coat, then stroll around for 20 or 30 minutes, enjoying the fresh air, and enjoying the little bit of people watching you are able to do as your feet carry you forward.

You have a meeting in the afternoon and are able to contribute a lot of quality thoughts to the proceedings. You're not entirely certain the company will actually use any of the ideas you presented, but it feels good to know you did your part to contribute to the growth and improvement of the company. You add more to your "to do" pile after the meeting, but you remind yourself, once more, that it's no big deal that the pile has grown so large. After all, there is only so much you can do each day. If you keep doing "what you can do each day," the pile will keep getting taken care of.

You leave work and sit in traffic again, but once more, it's not so bad. The evening is a great opportunity for you to spend a bit of time simply being quiet, no noise from the radio, no noise from the audiobook...nothing but you and your thoughts. You like to use this time to decompress from the day of work, and to reach a place of inner quiet and peace.

You stop at the gym on the way home and put in a quick workout, and by the time you arrive home you feel completely relaxed and ready to enjoy the evening. You sit down for dinner with your significant other (or with a friend you invited over for the evening), and you chat for about an hour, using this time to connect with one another.

After dinner, you sit outside and watch the night unfold around you. The sounds of the daytime hustle-and-bustle die away. The calm quiet of the night, and of this world that is so much bigger than any of us, pours over you, helping you relax...helping you feel happy and fulfilled.

Eventually, you go inside and pick up a book (or you play a card game with your significant other, or you turn on your favorite television show), and then you go to bed, feeling relaxed, and feeling excited about another weekday on the other side of sleep...

Later in this book, we are (of course) going to look at a picture of what it means to *LIVE BETTER* as someone who is in your 60s, 70s, 80s, or 90s, as someone past those "working years" and finally in that supposedly "golden age" of retirement. We are going to explore what a "full life" might look like for you. But, again, I feel it is important for people of all ages to understand what *LIVING BETTER* looks like even before retirement.

The example from the previous section, the example of you truly enjoying your weekdays and truly getting the most out of them, instead of just "making your way through them," gives us a foundation on which to build. The really awesome thing, if you are already retired, is that it is easier to make the transition to "thriving" over "surviving" in your situation, as you do not have to make the mental adjustment of "enjoying" work days (a task that, admittedly, is difficult for a lot of people to conquer).

If you are already retired, there are fewer obstacles in your path to making the most of each day. But, again, I truly feel that we gain a clearer picture of what *LIVING BETTER* looks like in retirement when we are able to see an example of what *LIVING BETTER* looks like even in those years throughout which it is more difficult to look forward to each day.

The mistake so many people make, throughout those working years, is that they get in the habit of always "getting through the day." So many people spend their entire life "looking forward" to something in the future, and because of this, they fail to ever truly enjoy the present.

If you are reading this book as someone still in your working years, realize that it is time for you to start *LIVING BETTER* right now. If you are able to start on this path now, you will eventually discover that you are in the habit of enjoying each moment of each day, instead of being in the habit of "waiting around for the good things to come." And as a result of this, by the time you retire, it will be easy for you to truly thrive in retirement as well.

And if you are already in your retirement years, it is time for you to start gaining a clear idea of what *LIVING BETTER* looks like, in order to reach a place where you are spending these years thriving, instead of spending these years simply surviving.

At this point, you may be asking why I am bringing up all this stuff about "enjoying life" and "living to the fullest." You may be wondering, "Isn't this supposed to be a book about being healthy and leading a longer, healthier life? Isn't this book supposed to help us continue living fully through our 80s and even into our 90s? Why is he talking about all this stuff about 'enjoying life'? How is that going to help me live a healthy life late into my 90s?"

If this is what you are wondering, I have good news for you:

We're getting to that right now.

In fact...we have been "getting to that" already, as everything in this chapter, everything about "what it looks like to live better," correlates directly with your health and your longevity.

Listen up.

This is one of the most important truths in this entire book. If you want to "thrive" instead of "survive," if you want to not only live into your 90s, but also enjoy life all along the way, this is going to be one of the most vital truths for you to grasp...

You ready? Here it is:

Everything in your body ties together.

Your emotional well-being has an impact on your physical health. Your mental well-being has an impact on your physical health. Your spiritual well-being has an impact on your physical health. Everything in your body ties together.

If you can grasp the principles behind LIVING BETTER, if you can reach a place where there is nothing you love more than to wake up each day and enjoy the adventure that awaits you, you will not only enjoy each day of your life a whole lot more...but you will also create the opportunity for you to have a lot more days ahead of you than you would otherwise have.

Everything in your body ties together.

This is why we have spent this chapter taking a close look at what it actually means to *LIVE BETTER*, what it actually means to truly, genuinely thrive...to truly, genuinely enjoy this gift of life, rather than just letting time pass and waiting for "the good things" to come our way at last.

Every day is a "good thing." Enjoy it. Because everything in your body ties together.

We're about to start digging deeper here. You ready? We're about to start looking at the ways in which all areas of your life tie into your health. It is time for you to start taking a holistic approach to your livelihood. It is time for you to understand the things you can do in order to ensure you are on the path to *LIVING LONGER AND BETTER...*

HOLISTIC OR HOKEY?

Does a holistic approach to health actually work?

"Holistic health." I know, it is something that gets a bad rap at times. It is a branch of medicine with a somewhat tarnished reputation. In fact, I would not be at all surprised if when you read those first two words, you sighed out loud. And you know what? I wouldn't blame you. Honestly. The "bad rap" and the "tarnished reputation" of holistic health are well deserved these days.

As you are surely aware, one of the greatest dreams most people have is that they would be able to make income independent of actual work, that they would be able to team up with some sort of miracle system that enables them to make money even when they are simply relaxing and enjoying life.

Furthermore, it is no secret that another one of the greatest dreams of most people is to be healthy (and, preferably, to not have to constantly visit a doctor in order to make sure this is the case).

These are probably things you have realized yourself. And if these are things you have realized yourself, you are not alone. There are also a lot of opportunistic entrepreneurs who have realized that A) Most people wish they could make money even while not working, and B) Most people want to be healthy...and as a result, these entrepreneurs have come up with "multi-level-marketing systems" that hock "miracle, holistic health" products.

People then sign up and pay a fee to be able to purchase the products at a discount...and then, they can get others to sign up underneath them. The more people they sign up (and the more people those they have signed up are able to pull on board as well), the more money they make in commission. Sounds great, right? People get to receive a discount on a "miracle, holistic health" product and they get to make money as others sign up to receive these same benefits.

The problem, however (as you are surely aware), is that most of these "miracle, holistic health" products do not actually work at all. These products have been cooked up by the entrepreneurs themselves (or by a creative team working with them), and rarely have any basis in scientific or medical fact. And while the entrepreneurs are making money hand-over-fist from their products, they are also chipping away at the reputation of genuine avenues of holistic health.

As you read this chapter, however (and as you read the principles from this chapter that we continue to carry throughout the rest of this book), realize that there is a side to holistic health that is absolutely true, and that is the simple fact; that (as stated at the end of the previous chapter) everything in your body ties together. When you take care of certain areas of your mental well-being, your physical well-being will be positively impacted as a result.

Regardless of what age you are, this is one of the most important concepts to understand if you have a desire to not only *LIVE BETTER*, but to also *LIVE LONGER.*

Are there hokey sides to holistic health? Of course there are. (Just ask the person trying to sell you the aromatic patch you can wear on your arm that will cure you of all your ailments.) But there is also a strong core of truth to the honest principles of holistic health.

When you take proper care of your body, your mind, your emotions, and your spirituality, you will find that living a long, healthy life is not nearly as elusive a dream as you maybe always imagined. In fact, that long, healthy life you desire is right there at your fingertips: all you have to do is take the right steps. All you have to do it take hold of all areas of your "self."

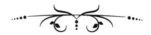

The Body

The primary determinate of longevity is mobility and exercise.

In my practice, one of the things I see most often is people in their 60s, 70s, 80s, and 90s who, quite frankly, have quit being active. Sure, they eat healthy. Sure, they get plenty of sleep and perhaps even keep a positive mental mindset. But when I ask them what they do to stay in shape, they look at me as if to say, "Doc, I'm 70 years old. Stay in shape? Come on, what do you want me to do, hit the gym or something?"

Honestly? The answer is yes, that's exactly what I want them to do.

Later in this chapter (after we touch on the basic ideas behind taking care of your body, your mind, your emotions, and your spirituality), I am going to give you a list of seven things you can do for your body, seven things, I'll venture so far as to say, you *should* be doing for your body in order to increase longevity, in order, that is to say, to help you LIVE LONGER AND BETTER. Before we get to that list, however, I want to talk a bit about the importance of taking care of your body.

The human body (as you know yourself, if you pause to think about it) is an incredible thing. Your body regulates itself in pretty much every way imaginable, keeping everything in balance, and fighting all the time to keep you healthy.

When you are young, of course, your body is resilient. Young people can eat poorly, fail to exercise, fail to remain active, and still be fairly healthy. Heck, there are plenty of young people who can eat poorly, fail to exercise, fail to remain active, and still have a great-looking body. But as you get older, that begins to change. Your body requires physical activity and stimulation in order to have the strength it needs to keep everything in balance.

One of the most important things we do at my practice is our comprehensive assessment of new patients. We look at a patient's nutritional status, making sure they are getting the proper calories, the proper proteins.

We look at their pharmacological status, checking to see if they are being overmedicated (you would be shocked to see just many of our patients are, in fact, being overmedicated). We do balance testing, strength testing, endurance testing. Why? Because all these things matter.

In the chapter of this book that deals directly with the overmedication problem among patients ages 60 to 90, we will look a bit more closely at exactly what the overmedication problem looks like, but a large part of it comes down to the fact that many doctors spend far more time and energy focusing on the problems they see, rather than focusing on what is causing the problems.

This leads to prescribing medication that will help cover up the symptoms, rather than looking for ways in which to eradicate the underlying illnesses and ailments themselves, something your body is far more equipped to do than most people (and even most doctors) give it credit for. For example: Did you know that muscle-strengthening exercises in arthritic body parts will cause roughly 50% of patients to get better? Not "muscle-strengthening exercises and medicine," but rather, just plain muscle-strengthening exercises alone.

That's right: the body is an amazing thing.

One of my favorite stories that illustrates the amazing value of this approach, of looking for ways in which illnesses and ailments can be eradicated, instead of simply prescribing medicine to cover up the illnesses and ailments in question, is about a 50-year-old female patient of mine who kept herself in remarkable shape (exercising regularly, taking her vitamin B12 shots, partaking in a diet high in fiber and getting a high dose of vitamin D), but who was nevertheless finding that her hair was thinning and her nails were becoming soft.

After exploring her dietary history, I realized that she was protein calorie malnourished. I immediately recommended that she start taking two scoops a day of bodybuilder's protein, and within a month her hair and nails had responded. Within six months, she was entirely back to normal.

The question you need to ask yourself, then, is this: "What am I doing to take care of my body?" Or rather: "What am I doing to take care of my body, in order to enable my body to take care of me?"

Have you ever visited your doctor and complained to him or her about the frequent shortness of breath you are dealing with? This is one of the most common complaints I receive in my practice. Oftentimes, these patients have visited other doctors, and these doctors have ordered an echocardiogram, a chest x-ray, and lung function tests. Then, everything comes back clean, and the doctors cannot figure it out.

These patients come to me and say, "I'll walk from the couch to the bathroom, and I'll be short of breath. What's wrong with me? The other doctors I visited aren't finding anything." They say, "Doc, I'm short of breath on a minimal amount of movement. What gives?"

Do you know what is usually wrong with these patients? Quite simply, that walk from the couch to the bathroom, or from the bedroom to the couch, is the only physical activity they have all day. We call it de-conditioning, and it is a very common complaint.

I've had patients before who use a wheelchair even though they do not need one. When I asked them why, they told me, "My back hurts when I stand."

The example I like to use in return is this:

As you know, I am a triathlete, but I do what are called "sprints," shorter triathlons that have, say, a three-mile run, a quarter-mile swim, and a 15-mile bike ride. That's what I train for.

But what would happen to me if I tried to go out and run a marathon (or even a half-marathon) tomorrow? I'll tell you what would happen: I'd spend about half of it in immense pain, and then I would probably be unable to finish. Why? Because I have not built up to a marathon or a half-marathon; I have not trained for that, but have instead trained for something that requires shorter, faster bursts.

The same is the case for individuals whose muscles ache when they use them.

Take, for example, someone who uses a wheelchair even though they do not need one. If one such individual chose to start doing some basic core exercises each day, it would not be long before they discovered that their back was not hurting as much when they stood. If, then, this individual started standing more often, they would soon discover that it is taking longer for their back to start giving them problems. In keeping this up, over time, this individual would ultimately realize that their back issues have gone away completely.

Your body is an amazing thing. Remember that. But also, remember: you need to give your body help if you want your body to help you in return.

If you want to *LIVE LONGER AND BETTER*, it's time to start taking an active interest in your body's fitness, and who knows, maybe one day soon we will be able to see each other at the next triathlon.

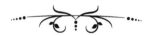

The Mind

Your brain is the command center for your entire body.

When you think of your brain, you probably think of it as "the part of my body that enables me to think." One thing many of us tend to forget, however, is that our conscious thoughts are not the only function of the brain (not by a long shot). Rather, our brain is working all the time, sending signals to every part of our body, telling our body what to do, how to feel, how to act and react. Our brain is the command center of our entire body.

Once you think about this, then, it can really start to cause you to wonder, "What am I doing to keep my brain in good shape?"

What are you doing to keep your mind sharp?

One of the greatest issues people end up dealing with as they advance in years is that their brain begins to deteriorate. Their mind starts to slip. In fact, this tends to be one of the greatest fears among those who are getting older: Fear of dementia, fear of memory loss, fear of Alzheimer's...fear of being incapable of taking care of yourself mentally. It's a scary thought, I know. But let me ask you this:

How many 70-year-olds or 80-year-olds do you see who never retired, who are in their 70s or even in their 80s, but have nevertheless chosen to work every day, just as they had for decades before, and who have dementia?

You would be hard-pressed to find someone in their 70s or 80s who is still working, and who has dementia.

On the other hand, those who retire are far more likely to deal with mental deficiencies over time. The reason for this? It's simple, really: In the same way many people ages 60 and up have stopped remaining physically active, many individuals quit keeping themselves "mentally active" after they retire. As described earlier in this book: Most days look pretty much the same, wake up, sit down in the recliner or on the couch, turn on the television, and sit there until the day ends.

What would your body look like if you sat perfectly still and ate nothing but junk food every single day? Well, this is what a person is doing to their mind when they sit in front of a television all day. They are feeding their mind nothing but "junk food," and they are, for the most part, remaining entirely unengaged in regards to mental stimulation.

The brain begins to lose its "strength," because it is not being "exercised." The brain, then, becomes less able to stay sharp in such areas as memory, problem-solving, communication, retention, and so on. Furthermore, the brain begins to lose its ability to direct your body as effectively as it should.

Those who continue working tend to remain physically active, socially connected, and mentally challenged, all of which are known to prevent mental decline. Furthermore, those who engage in a consistent exercise routine reduce their risk of developing age-related dementia. How much of a difference can quality exercise lower your risk of dementia? By as much as 45%.[1]

Remember: your brain is the command center for your entire body. If you allow your brain to remain dormant for days at a time, then, how can you expect it to be sharp when you need it to be sharp?

As with "the body," you will find a list at the end of this chapter of things you should be doing in order to keep your mind sharp. "Living better," after all, certainly means living with a fully-functioning brain. And this means that it is time for you to start doing your part to ensure your brain is functioning as well as it possibly can.

---

[1] "Exercise to Prevent Dementia," Alzheimers.org. uk. Retrieved January 20, 2015. From http://www.alzheimers. org.uk/site/scripts/documents_info. php?documentID =2211&pageNumber=7

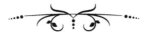

Emotions

Are you excited about life, or are you simply passing through each day?

I'll share a secret with you (or...perhaps it is not so much of a secret; perhaps this is something you could guess quite easily yourself, or is even something you have experienced first-hand). The secret is this:

Most medical doctors are extremely logical individuals.

As doctors, we deal in concrete terms; in the results of arduous scientific and medical research, and in quantifiable results. As doctors, we are trained to examine cause and effect as best we can...determining what elements are present (or "out of order") in the body, and are therefore causing the problems individuals are dealing with, in order for us to then determine what needs to be done to fix said problems. As doctors, we deal in test results and data so frequently that many of my peers end up minimizing the importance of, or even altogether forgetting about, emotions.

Emotions, after all, are not something that can be medically tested; they are not something that can be quantifiably measured and charted. Emotions, by their very nature, are abstract, at their core. In fact, emotions are formless, and are only given form by the names we as a society have ascribed to each particular emotion, and because of this, many doctors overlook the importance of emotions.

And, of course, because many patients trust their doctor to be their most reliable source of medical knowledge and advice, and because most doctors never talk about emotions in the first place, most individuals rarely think of the manner in which their emotions correlate to their health.

As a result of this, I feel that one of the things many of us fail to really consider is the manner in which negative thoughts and emotions affect our body's ability to take care of itself...our body's ability, I will go so far as to say, to heal itself.

Think about it. This is something most doctors and patients alike fail to ponder as often as they should: The greatest healing tool in the modern world is still our very own body.

Everything in your body is engineered to help you both prevent diseases and fight diseases that happen to come upon you. As we touched on in the last section, of course, your brain is the command center for your entire body, and part of the job your brain undertakes in keeping you healthy is that it instructs your body to take care of itself and heal itself in a myriad of ways.

What happens, then, when your mind is feeling bogged down with negative thoughts and emotions? What happens, in fact, when your emotions are leading your mind to think negatively about your health and your body?

Did you catch that?

That is one of the most important things you will read in this book, one of the most important thoughts for you to pause and ponder. I'll go ahead and repeat it:

What happens when your emotions are leading your mind to think negatively about your health and your body?

When your body heals itself, this is part of the natural course according to the design of your body... but in order for your body to take the steps it must take in order to heal itself, your brain must instruct it to do so. So what makes you think your brain is instructing your body to heal itself when you are allowing your brain to think nothing but negative thoughts?

No, it may not be quantifiable. It may not be something on which we can collect data, something we can test medically, scientifically...but this does not make it any less true. And, in fact, the dismissive attitude so many doctors take toward a patient's emotional state actually makes the threat of our negative emotions even greater, as so few patients ever stop to consider this as an area they need to pay attention to.

How do we make sure we are maintaining a positive outlook? The first step, quite simply, is to understand how important it really is to be positive.

If you stop to think about it, you already know that when you feel positive, you feel practically indestructible. According to Barbara Fredrickson's "broaden and build" theory[2], if we cultivate those

---

[2] "The Broaden-and-Build Theory of Positive Emotions." Wikipedia.org. Retrieved February 24, 2015 from www.wikipedia.org/wiki/Broaden-and-build.

positive feelings enough, we begin to build an emotional reserve to draw upon when we are at a low point. Think about it.

If you could make your positive feelings last longer, more people would want to be around you, and this would lead to more resilient social connections. This is a lesson you need to start learning. When something inspiring or uplifting happens, one way to make it last longer is by sharing it with other people.

Another way to remain positive is by relishing the moment as long as you can. As you make a concerted effort to linger in positive emotions, it will become easier for you to store these emotions for future retrieval. Start being intentional with your positive emotions; share them with others, linger on them, build memories about them, think about them, and save them deep in your positive memory bank.

Don't take for granted positive or joyful moments. Instead, take pride in what you have obtained, congratulate yourself, tell yourself, "You did a good job." Even small things, a completed exercise routine, for instance, can be turned into positive memories that can be drawn on later. These positive memories will build and reinforce themselves and will help you do more next time.

One of the best examples in my personal life of positive thinking took place around a natural phenomenon that many of us have dealt with; thinning hair. In spite of the fact that this is a completely healthy and natural occurrence, most of us who have experienced thinning hair know that it can have a negative emotional impact. Am I right? (I'll answer that for you: Of course I am.)

But when I was younger and started experiencing thinning hair myself, I made a conscious decision that I would not allow something over which I had no control to negatively affect my emotional well-being or my life.

Every time I felt compromised by my hair situation, I would immediately switch my thoughts to something positive. What did my "positive thought" look like? I would think of a Caribbean beach scene that I had experienced previously. What's more positive than that? Instead of sitting with thoughts about my thinning hair, I was escaping to a beautiful beach where I was playing Frisbee with an attractive girl and other friends.

Before I knew it, the negative thoughts would be gone, and it wasn't long before I felt that I was entirely well adjusted to my situation, to a point where I no longer felt despair or concerns when I considered my thinning hair.

Another way to tap into a more positive emotional state and to reduce stress at the same time is through meditation. A University of Wisconsin health study revealed increased electrical activity in the regions of the brain that tend to be more active in optimistic people after a course in meditation training. Of course, we will be getting to some thoughts on spirituality and meditation here in just a bit, but it is important for you to realize just how much this can tie into a positive emotional state.

If you are dealing with a negative emotional state, it is time to start figuring out ways in which to turn it around. You may not believe me right now, as you read this, but once you test the veracity of this section for yourself, you will be shocked by the results. You know how I know? I know because I see it all the time.

Patients who complain about how nothing goes right, about how they can't get healthy, about how they are doomed to deal with medical issues for the rest of their lives, generally tend to find that these words of theirs come true, these negative things they are expecting to happen do, in fact, continue to happen.

But on the other hand, those individuals who keep a positive outlook toward their body, their health, and their life, even when it seems, on the surface, that things are not going well in one (or even all) of these areas, always tend to see improvements more quickly than expected, and always deal with far fewer problems.

Have you paused lately to assess your emotional state? Have you asked yourself if you are happy, content, satisfied? Are you excited about life, or are you simply passing through each day? Are you staying positive? Are you living for something...or are you instead just "living"?

Your brain is the command center for your entire body...

...and your emotions dictate, to a large extent, the effectiveness of your brain.

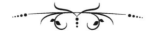

Spirituality

With a greater level of inner peace comes a greater level of health, happiness, and fulfillment.

If it is true that many doctors do not pause as much as they should to think about emotions and the role emotions play in our body's ability to properly heal itself. It is just as true that many doctors do not pause as much as they should to think about the manner in which spirituality ties into an individual's emotional state.

Now, when I speak of spirituality, I do so from my place as a devout Christian, but I also speak to you on this topic without pigeonholing spirituality into one specific religious box. If you are into spirituality, but are not a Christian, everything I say here applies to you as well. And even if you are agnostic or downright atheistic, everything I speak of in this section on spirituality applies to you.

After all, even those who do not believe in a higher power will tend to agree that there is something much greater to the world, and to life, than simply our individual lives. And whether you believe this "something greater" to be a Creator, or to be the Earth itself, or to be our collective consciousness, or to be any of a number of other things, there are ways in which the benefits of "spirituality" can be accessed by you, can, that is to say, be accessed by all.

One of the major elements of spirituality that causes it to tie into the health of our bodies is the inner peace that tends to come alongside a firm belief in, and indulgence in, a spiritual side to the world. For myself, it is through daily prayer that I am able to achieve a sense of peace and strength, and I know that this peace and strength carries over to my emotions, and therefore to my body's ability to properly heal and take care of itself.

For others, I know, meditation is a powerful tool for reaching a place of peace and assurance in life and in the world around them.

And even if "prayer" and "meditation" are ideas that do not reconcile with the logical side of your mind, just plain quiet can go a long way toward creating a sense of inner peace. Yes, quiet...which is something many of us, sadly, are wholly unfamiliar with.

While some may deem all this talk of "meditation" to be, as the title of this chapter suggests, a bit "hokey," many of these same people fail to realize that the words "meditation," "medicine," and "medication" all share the same Latin roots: *medicus* (which means "to cure") and *mederi* (which means "to heal"). Meditation allows us to disengage our conscious mind in order to begin healing and to achieve a positive atmosphere for our body to rest.

As we begin to disengage our lives from the surrounding environment, our pulse, blood pressure, and breathing all decrease, along with pain and anxiety. Furthermore, exercise tolerance and maximum workload increase. By practicing meditation, you give yourself the power to change your attitude and beliefs, as well as your reactions to the environment around you, thereby influencing your physical, mental, social, and spiritual well-being.

Why is this important? Because we live in a stressful world. We can often find ourselves in a "fight or flight" composure, but meditation is the opposite; it allows us to rest and puts us in a situation where we will not have the need for "fight or flight."

Believe it or not, I actually engage in meditation with many of my patients. At the end of a visit to my office, I will often say a prayer with my patient. As a doctor practicing in the southern part of the country, I have found that a moment of prayer with their doctor is very much welcomed and appreciated by most patients, including those of varying faiths. During this short time of prayer, my patient and I are ultimately engaging in meditation together; invariably, I get a smile and a "Thank you" for the positive impact this small gesture has on them.

If you think that the idea of "meditation" sounds overwhelming, realize that this is not at all the case. Anyone can practice meditation (this includes you), and best of all, it doesn't cost any money. You can practice prayer and meditation anywhere. I personally enjoy praying in the morning or while I am biking, running, and swimming, as this enables me to keep the worries of a busy life at bay during my free time, which gives me double benefits of both exercising my body and eliminating stress.

Not only can meditation help you enjoy "your own time" more, but current research also suggests that many symptoms associated with anxiety disorders, asthma, cancer, depression, heart disease, high blood pressure, pain, and sleep problems can all be improved with prayer and meditation.

There is a lot written about various types of meditation, but in my experience, quality meditation starts with finding a quiet setting where you can learn how to breathe in a relaxed manner as you focus your attention on something positive (in my case, I focus my attention on something related to God, but as I stated earlier, even someone who is non-religious can find something positive and pleasant on which to focus... something greater than their own self). A comfortable position is also very much recommended; I used to pray on my knees, but that is not sustainable for a long period of time. Nowadays, I choose to lie down with a pillow under my head (out of bed, in order to prevent falling asleep).

Because of the busy nature of the lives so many of us lead, most of us go through our working years with very little downtime. And then, when we do have downtime, we use it in conversation with others, or with our nose in a book, or with the radio playing or the television going or our thoughts chasing themselves in circles through our brain. What many of us do not pause to indulge in, and this even goes for retired individuals who have more time on their hands with that 40-hour work week behind them forever, is that precious gift of absolute stillness.

Take some time each day to turn off your brain, even just for five minutes. Get in the habit of putting your mind to rest, just for a bit. Sit perfectly still. Think about nothing. When your thoughts try to rise up, push them back down. It may sound difficult, and honestly, for most people, it is even more difficult than it sounds. We are so unused to giving our minds a break, so unused to sitting in true stillness and silence, that we do not even know how to actually do this.

As we sit in stillness and attempted silence, most of us last about 15 seconds before our thoughts rise up uninvited and start bouncing around the inside of our head. But as with anything, practice makes perfect. And once you reach that point where you can finally sit perfectly still for five minutes (or, eventually, for 10 minutes, or 15 minutes) without moving, without thinking (without worrying and working and wandering mentally), once you reach that place from which you can truly and wholly indulge in stillness and silence, you will begin to experience the rejuvenating effects such stillness and silence can have.

Yes, prayer and meditation take practice; in the beginning, your busy mind will fight hard to remain at rest, but as you gain experience, you will begin to gain the upper hand on these intruding streams of jumbled (and usually stressful) thoughts.

Of course, silence is not the only means of achieving inner peace through spirituality. If you are a Christian, or if you are a Muslim, or if you are a Buddhist, or if you adhere to any other form of organized religion or spirituality, one of the most important things I can suggest that you do is that you make sure you are following the principles of your religion in more than name alone. When you actually take the time to connect with a higher power, you will realize a much greater level of peace than you have ever experienced before. And, of course, with a greater level of inner peace comes a greater level of health, happiness, fulfillment, and life.

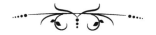

7 Keys to *LIVING LONGER AND BETTER:*

<u>Body</u>

1.   Core exercises

"Abs: they're just for looks, right?" Absolutely not. In fact, there are plenty of reasons beyond "looks" why you should make sure you are focusing on your core... reasons that actually apply to you as a 60-year-old, 70-year-old, 80-year-old, or 90-year-old.

Stabilize lower back: If you have been dealing with lower back pain, one of the main causes for this may be the weakened state of your core muscles. Once you get your core muscles to the place where they need to be, you will find that you are dealing with far fewer lower back issues.

The lower back is so important that I actually want to linger on it a moment longer and make sure you understand exactly *how* and *why* it is so important to stabilize your lower back. You see, your spine is surrounded by muscles, the back muscles themselves, which support the back of the spine, and the abdominal muscles, which support the front of the spine.

When you strengthen the muscles surrounding the front and back of the spine, you prevent the development of arthritis in the spine. Arthritis, in most cases, is really just an overgrowth of bone tissue in response to abnormal stress. And one of the best ways to prevent abnormal stress is by strengthening our muscles. If we strengthen the back muscles as well as the abdominal muscles, this will support the spine, and will prevent arthritis, pain, and pressure on nerves.

This is important to understand, as "back pain" is one of the most common complaints I see in my office, and it is one of the easiest to prevent and treat with simple exercise. Even sciatica, when the pain starts to go down the back of the legs, is simply the cause of an arthritic back with overgrowth of bone pressing upon the nerve.

All of this could be avoided with a strong core, including back and abdominal muscles. Before I do any exercise, I always begin each session by stretching my legs and then going right to exercises for my abs and back. I do this to make sure this most important portion of my workout never, ever gets missed or overlooked.

Improve balance and coordination: One of the greatest fears many people have as they get older is that they will one day fall when no one is around, and will be stuck on the floor, unable to get up. Of course, the reason this is "one of the greatest fears" many people have as they get older is because this is something that actually happens to people, time and time again. We hear about it...and then, we get fearful that this could happen to us. And yes, this is a big deal.

More than 30% of people over 65 fall each year, and when you fall when you are 80 and break a hip, the chances of dying within one year get close to 40%. In fact, 90% of all hip fractures occur in people over 60, and once you become fearful of falling, there is a vicious, downward cycle in which you tend to get up less because of this fear, which leads to your muscles weakening...which leads to a higher likelihood of falling more.

Many doctors in the field talk about self-efficacy, in other words, self-confidence, and a very easy way to gain confidence is by simply practicing the things you know will work. For example, strengthening the core muscles. One of the best ways to improve balance and coordination, and to therefore prevent one of those falls from occurring, is by simply strengthening your core muscles.

Promote better breathing: When your core is strong, you are far less likely to encounter difficulties breathing. When, on the other hand, you fail to properly strengthen and maintain your core muscles, you will be at a heightened risk for dealing with respiratory issues.

Make it easier to do other physical activities: When you have a strong core, nearly every other physical activity will be made easier. As you age and deal with what would otherwise be a worrisome time health-wise, there is very little that feels better than having a strong core and knowing that this is making all other areas of physical activity easier as a result.

When you hear the recommendation that you should "focus on your core," it may seem as though this is not as important as the person making the suggestion is making it sound. But truth be told, strengthening your core is about the most important thing you can do to promote strength and health in the rest of your body.

2. Walking

As you grow older, it becomes increasingly important that you keep your body active, but this does not have to mean strenuous activity. In fact, simply walking can work wonders on your overall health. When you are walking on a daily basis (walking, that is, further than the distance from your bedroom to your couch), you will keep your body in the habit of being physically active, and this will ultimately result in your body continuing to "work to take care of itself" in the manner it is supposed to.

If you live in a temperate climate, the option of walking outdoors obviously makes it very easy to ensure you are partaking in this activity each and every day, but even if you live in an area that has inclement weather during parts of the year (either too hot in the summer, or too cold in the winter), one option to consider is walking at the mall.

If you visit the mall around the time it first opens, you will not only find that the entire building is not yet busy and crowded, but you will also find that there are plenty of others just like you who are using this "indoor track" to do their daily walking.

"But Doc, how important is walking, really?" I'm glad you asked. Men in the Honolulu heart study who walked two miles a day were able to reduce the risk of death by half, while walking also helped to prevent weight gain and reduced the risk of breast and colon cancer.

There was also a study conducted by the National Council on Aging that discovered that those who walked 45 minutes each day reduced the risk of stroke, heart disease, and diabetes, while also experiencing a boost in brain power and thinking skills. Walking also improves mood and helps prevent erectile dysfunction. So, how important is walking, really? Extremely important.

3.   Stretching

Have you ever complained about your body feeling "tight"? Not just a particular muscle, either, but your body as a whole? This is a common complaint as people get older, but many people fail to realize that the solution to this problem can be as simple as stretching. By keeping your body limber and well stretched, you will prevent the discomfort that comes from a body that feels "tight," and you will help your body remain in an optimal position for effectively taking care of itself.

When you stretch, it will be important that you focus on each specific part of your body, doing stretches that target all areas of your legs, that target your back, and that target your arms. Stretching is one of the easiest (and most relaxing.) things you can do for your body, and it will also go a long way toward ensuring that your body continues to function as it is supposed to function.

4. Biking

Biking is one of the best full-body workouts in which you can partake, as biking not only works out your legs, but it also provides a workout for your core and even for your arm muscles. Biking also puts you in a position to keep your sense of balance sharp, while helping you engage in an all-important cardiovascular workout.

One of the best examples I received of the positive impact of biking came when I went on a recent ski trip. Of course, I work hard to keep myself in good shape, but I could tell a significant difference in my legs on the slopes from the time I had spent biking.

Biking makes us use short bursts of high-intensity energy to raise the heart rate similar to skiing, and I was therefore pleasantly surprised to discover how well I tolerated my ski trip. And realize: you do not need to bike outdoors all the time; a stationary bike can be great regardless of the weather or location, and will allow you to adjust settings for varying levels on intensity.

While biking does not need to be part of your daily routine, it is certainly something you should make an effort to do from time to time...and, of course, if you wanted to make biking part of your daily routine, this would certainly not be a bad thing.

5. Swimming

One of the best things about swimming is that, in addition to being another tremendous full-body workout, it is a low-impact workout, meaning that you will be far less likely to deal with sore joints from your excursions into the pool than you would be after running or engaging in a similarly high-impact workout.

Swimming is the most aerobic exercise available, and it uses more muscle groups than any other exercise. It is also extremely refreshing, as gravity puts less stress and pressure on the large, weight-bearing joints (hips, knees, ankles, etc.). If arthritis caused by years of weight-bearing exercise is an issue for you, swimming is a great alternative.

Furthermore, swimming can be a great workout if you are injured, as an injured individual will be able to put on a flotation belt and run in water as if they were running online, but without pressure on the joints.

If you have a pool at your own house, of course, it will be easy for you to add "swimming" to your routine of staying active and taking care of your body, but even if you do not have a pool, realize that there are plenty of places where you can pay a small membership fee and have access to a pool.

Regardless of whether you choose to engage in something organized, such as water aerobics, or choose to instead use your pool time to simply swim a few laps, you should definitely make sure you are getting into a pool on a regular basis.

6. Strength training

Look, I don't expect you to go to the gym at the age of 70 and bench press 300 pounds, and you should not expect to do this, either. As you move into your 60s, 70s, 80s, and 90s, the idea of "building muscle," of "bulking up" as you hit the gym, can safely go out of the window. This does not mean, however, that you should not be lifting weights or taking part in other activities intentionally designed to strengthen your muscles.

After all, your muscles are ultimately going to be the tools your body uses in order to help you move around effectively for as long as you are alive. By placing an emphasis on muscle strengthening, you will ensure that you are putting yourself in a position to move around and function with little to no issues.

In order to continually keep your muscles strong and healthy, you should be focusing on low-impact workouts, generally aiming for lower weights and higher repetitions. When you engage in such workouts, you will keep your muscles strong and healthy without putting unnecessary wear and tear on them, thereby ensuring that you are getting the most out of your workouts.

I recommend compound exercises that involve groups of muscles, rather than isolating one specific muscle on which to focus. Pull-ups, squats, and bench press are all considered compound exercises, and are all-beneficial for the way in which they are able to spread the stress of the exercise over many muscles and cause the entire body to work together.

With compound exercises, you are doing more total work in a short amount of time, and this work will stimulate the muscles and bones to gain strength in more parts of the body. And as you increase the weight, your frame and skeleton will increase accordingly to match the stress placed upon them. Under these circumstances, you will mitigate your risk of osteoporosis (thinning of the bones), as well as the risk of arthritis, and, of course, the risk of injuries during everyday life.

7.   Be INTENTIONAL with your body

How often do you think about your body and the way you are treating it? Sure, there might be times when you think about your body and the "way it is treating you," but most people fail to really pause and think about how they are treating their body.

As you move through life, as you move through each day, you should always be thinking, in the back of your mind, about the impact your decisions are having on your body. Are you giving your body the right foods? Are you getting a proper amount of sleep? Are you staying active, treating your body well so that your body can treat you well in return? As you move through your day, ask yourself how you are treating your body. Be INTENTIONAL about this. Trust me, it's worth it. After all, when you take care of your body, your body will ultimately take care of you.

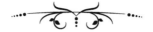

7 Keys to *LIVING LONGER AND BETTER:*

<u>Mind</u>

1.   Read for pleasure

Surely, you've heard people say it before when someone brings up a novel they particularly enjoyed... you've heard a response that goes something like this: "I only read books I can learn from." There are a lot of people who take this approach to fiction reading, basically implying that reading novels is a waste of time, and that if they are going to read, they are going to use that time to read something "important," something they can learn from, or something that will help them further their own self.

And yet, most people who take this approach toward fiction reading nevertheless spend a decent chunk of time each week watching television shows or movies or sports. When it comes down to it, of course, reading "for pleasure" or "for fun" is not as productive as reading "to learn"...but with that said, reading "for pleasure" is far more productive than watching television shows or sports "for pleasure."

When you read, your mind is automatically being kept mentally engaged, essentially, your mind is being kept "sharp," and this is true regardless of whether you are reading "for pleasure" or "to learn."

If reading is already a favorite activity of yours, realize that it is quite a beneficial activity as well. And if you have strayed away from fiction reading for one reason or another but still indulge in other forms of entertainment (forms of entertainment that fail to sharpen your mind.), it is time for you to pick up a few good books and spend some time experiencing the joy of reading. After all, we all know that "the book is always better than the movie," right? And even beyond the "enjoyment factor," there is a real benefit to be gained from reading over processing images or speech when watching a movie.

The neuroscience guys teach us that, just like the muscles, the brain benefits from a good workout, so reading is just what the doctor ordered as a good workout for your brain. Instead of just processing images and speech by watching television or a movie, you will be engaging many parts of your brain when you read. And just like lifting weights, you will be using multiple "muscle groups" in your brain by reading.

Just as a bench press helps to work out your biceps, shoulders, chest, back, and ab muscles, what we referred to before as a "compound exercise," reading compounds the number of areas of the brain being involved, which multiplies the benefits of this brain-stimulating activity.

Our intelligence is called into action when we read, and we are forced into greater concentration as we imagine what is going on in the story, all of which helps to sharpen the memory and keep it nimble and strong, even as we age.

2. Read to learn

Of course, all that talk about how great it is to read for pleasure is not intended to take away from how tremendously beneficial it can also be to read for the purpose of learning. "Continuing education" is one of the best ways to ensure that your mind is as sharp as it can possibly be, and "continuing education" does not have to mean formal classes.

One of the best ways to "continue education" is by reading for the purpose of learning, as this will help you to continually keep your mind moving forward, and to "exercise" your brain to an extensive degree.

Many people find that the best way to "read for learning" is to settle on a topic about which they are interested in learning as much as they can. By doing this, you will create a purpose to your learning, as you will be able to ultimately make a list of all the books you want to read in that particular area of learning (a much better approach than simply picking up random books on random topics, which can leave you feeling aimless and even bored with the "reading for learning" you are doing).

By the time you have made your way through all the books you are wanting to read in a particular area of focus, you will likely have two or three new "areas of focus" you are wanting to study next, and you will be able to move forward to a new area of focus, keeping the mental momentum going, and keeping your mind as sharp as you want it to be.

3.   Remain social

Social interactions are extremely important, especially as you get older. Not only are we nurtured, emotionally, by our rewarding interactions with others, but we are also mentally stimulated by time spent with friends. By having friends with whom you can share quality conversation, you will keep your mind engaged and sharp.

What's more, having friends with whom you regularly spend time is a big part of *LIVING BETTER*, making sure you are "thriving" and truly enjoying this wonderful stage of life, instead of simply "surviving" and waiting for time to pass.

Oftentimes, it will be up to you to be "intentional" about spending time with those individuals with whom you are close. Far too often, people of all ages never spend as much time around their friends as they would like, simply because most of us do a poor job planning events and get-togethers.

A great way to combat this is to have a particular day of the week or month on which you always get together with a certain friend or group of friends. By doing this, you will ensure that you are regularly seeing the people it is important for you to see. (Furthermore, realize that you can have several friends or several groups of friends with whom you have regular days or evenings planned, putting you in a position where your calendar each month is full of social outlets even before anything "spontaneous" has been planned for the month.)

And realize: this truly is important. According to the University of Michigan, remaining social and talking for just 10 minutes a day to another person can improve memory and mental performance[3]. Socializing can be just as effective as the more traditional mental exercises (crossword puzzles, memory games, etc.).

We can also delay memory loss as we age by having an active social life, according to the Harvard School of Public Health[4]. Being social makes us mentally engaged in a way that is distinct from completing games and puzzles, so go out, and get engaged in a network of friends. Volunteer at church, join a book club, get involved in your community, do something to connect with others around you.

4. Puzzle games (yes, they really work.)

This is such an obvious suggestion that it often goes overlooked. In fact, it is such an obvious suggestion that many people see it as somewhat silly. "Really," they think, "you want me to play puzzle games and

---

[3] "Ten minutes of talking has a mental payoff." Retrieved January 27, 2015 from http://www.nsf.gov/mobile/news/news_summ.jsp?cntn_id=110690&org=SBE&from=new

[4] Ertel, Karen A.; Glymour, M. Maria; Berkman, Lisa F. "Effects of Social Integration on Preserving Memory Function in a Nationally Representative US Elderly Population." Retrieved on September 3, 2015 from http://www.ncbi.nlm.nih.gov/pmc/articles/PMC2424091/

memory games on the computer?" But as silly as it can seem at times, it truly does work.

"Synapse formation" in the brain (what many people refer to as "connections" in the brain, or even "bridges" in the brain) is an extremely important part of maintaining and improving brain function, and any time you engage your brain in problem-solving activities, new synapses are formed. This leads to a stronger and sharper brain, which leads to a longer and better life.

If you are the kind of person who enjoys a challenge in the form of puzzles, anything from jigsaw puzzles to Sudoku to computer games geared toward problem solving can be a great way to enjoy an hour or two of an afternoon.

Even if this is not your idea of "fun," you should make an effort to incorporate these activities into your week, intentionally spending a bit of time with "synapse formation" through games that test and strengthen your memory and/or problem-solving abilities, as this will go a long way toward keeping your mind sharp and alert.

5.   Use all your senses

Our senses are an interesting contributor to the sharpness of our minds, namely because senses are a big part of memory. Certain smells, for example, can evoke certain memories; certain sounds can bring up emotions connected to those sounds; the feel of certain items can awaken memories that have been dormant for years. However, as with anything in our bodies, our senses can become dull if we are not putting them to use.

Of course, the idea of purposing to "use all five of your senses" on a regular basis goes by the wayside if you are taking care of the other things you should be taking care of in order to *LIVE LONGER AND BETTER* (that is to say: if you are truly living life and "thriving," you will be engaging with the world using all five of your senses anyway, and will not have to go out of your way to do so intentionally), but nevertheless, this is something worth being cognizant of in your own life. Keep your senses active and engaged, and they will continue to repay you with the ways in which they help keep your memory sharp.

6.   Prioritize the way you are using your brain

Your brain does not have infinite space. Have you ever thought of that before? And when it comes down to it, the less you have to add to your brain, the more optimally your brain will be able to function. How, then, do you make sure you are not adding unnecessary items to your brain? It's simple: keep your life well organized.

With a well-organized life, you will be able to effectively siphon thoughts out of your brain, leaving your mind less cluttered, and creating more room for the day-to-day functions in which your mind needs to engage in order for you to have an optimal life.

For example, set your keys and your wallet in the same place every day, so you are never left trying to remember where you left them. Keep a calendar that has upcoming events written on it, and that has important dates clearly marked (grandchildren's birthdays, holidays, commitments, etc.).

Set your computer to remember all passwords, and then keep your passwords hidden away in a notebook in case you ever need them. Store phone numbers in your phone, and store addresses in an address book or on your computer. Make notes in advance that remind you of the date on which you need to change the oil in your car or change the filters in your air conditioning unit.

The less "maintenance" you have to use your mind for, the freer your mind will be to focus on things that are ultimately far more important, and the sharper you will find you are keeping your mind as a result.

7. Be *INTENTIONAL* with your mind

Naturally, "being intentional" is, once more, the seventh and final point. How are you using your mind? What are you actively doing each day in order to ensure your mind is in the best possible position to take care of you? Are you feeding your mind "junk food," or are you taking steps each and every day to make your mind as sharp and clear as it can possibly be?

The more intentional you are with each and every day, considering the effects that even your casual actions will have on your mind, and consequently staying away from actions that will dull your mind, while gravitating toward actions that will sharpen your mind, the more you will discover you are having no problems relying on your mind for everything from memory to fresh thoughts to the all-important direction your body receives from your mind every second of every day.

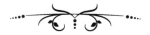

7 Keys to *LIVING LONGER AND BETTER*

<u>Emotions</u>

1. Avoid stress

You may have heard it said before; "stress is the silent killer." Of course, this may sound dramatic (and sure, it is a bit dramatic), but this statement is also rooted firmly in truth. When you are dealing with stress, you will not only be negatively affecting your emotions, but will also be negatively affecting everything from your immune system to your body's ability to properly manage itself in a day-to-day manner.

Of course, saying that you should "avoid stress" is all well and good, right? But as we all know, actually following through with this can be far more difficult. If you find that you deal with stress on a regular basis, here are a few tips that will help you to manage stress more effectively:

Identify the source of your stress: When you are able to figure out what is causing your stress, you will be able to then determine what (if anything) you can do to fix this problem. If the problem is something you can fix yourself, make a list of the action steps you can take in order to fix it. And if the problem is something that is outside of your control, start practicing an approach to this problem that basically says, "Hey, there is nothing I can do about it, so there is no reason for me to worry about it."

Learn to relax: In the same way you should be striving to achieve the sort of inner peace that often comes with spirituality, you should also be striving to intentionally relax. Of course, for some of us, "relaxing" is not an issue, but there are many of us who actually thrive off high-pressure situations. When these high-pressure situations no longer exist, (for example, when you are retired and no longer have deadlines to meet and pressing tasks to take care of), such individuals will turn non-issues into "high-pressure situations."

This is a very negative cycle, and leads to additional stress, which leads to a poor emotional state and a negative impact on your body. Remember: it is okay to relax. If this is something that does not come naturally to you, you need to train yourself to take the time to relax every now and then.

Exercise: Yes, I know, the last thing you probably feel like doing when you are feeling stressed is a bit of exercise (especially if you have not been exercising for years, and are just now making a resolution to get back on track with your physical fitness). But as unappealing as it may sound in the moment to "workout" or "exercise" when you are stressed, exercise is actually a tremendous way to enable your body to effectively manage stress.

When you workout, your body releases endorphins, which are essentially the "feel-good" neurotransmitters in your body. Furthermore, people often find that they are able to "intentionally trick themselves" into exercising. What do I mean by "intentionally tricking yourself?"

Basically, give yourself a low time limit of how long your workout will last. Say, "Sure, I don't feel like working out, but I will work out for 15 minutes." By the time you are 15 minutes into your workout, you will probably be feeling good enough that you will want to keep going.

Know what you love doing: One thing that causes people to get stressed and overwhelmed is that they spend far too much time doing things they do not actually enjoy. This is another habit many of us pick up during our working years, as a great majority of the population is comprised of individuals who convince themselves they do not like what they do for work (studies say that only 10% of working people enjoy what they do for a living), and who then, of course, spend the bulk of their week doing this "thing they do not enjoy doing." This ends up carrying over into retirement for many people, as they have gotten so used to "doing something they do not enjoy" with the bulk of their time, and they end up having a difficult time making the adjustment to a life of actually doing what they enjoy.

Once you are able to identify the things in life you truly enjoy, the things you would genuinely love to spend your time doing, you will be able to engage in these things as often as possible, which will ultimately cause you to feel more fulfilled in life, and will help to minimize the stress you deal with. (And if you are still in the working world and do not enjoy what you do for a living, try this solution: commit to giving it 110%. Most people find that this makes those around them happy, including their superiors, which then leads to a subsequent increase in job satisfaction.)

Spend time with people you enjoy being around: The more time you spend around people you love, people you truly enjoy, the more relaxed you will feel, and the less stress you will end up dealing with in your everyday life. While this may sound obvious, the actual fact of the matter is that most people would not even be able to say with absolute certainty who they would classify as the "people they enjoy being around."

Take the time to become aware of exactly who you do and do not enjoy being around, and then attempt to limit your exposure to those you do not enjoy being around (as much as it is possible to limit your exposure, that is), and make a concerted effort to spend time around those you enjoy being around. This will ultimately go a long way toward minimizing the amount of stress you deal with on a daily basis.

2.   Think in positives

There are two specific things I mean when I suggest that you "think in positives." Firstly, I mean that you should be thinking positive thoughts. This one is simple, right? (At least, it should be.) After all, the more positive-minded you are, the likelier it will always be that positive outcomes occur in your life. The other way in which I mean that you should "think in positives," however, is a way many people do not ever think of, and that is that when you are trying to do something differently in your life, you should always state what you wish to do, rather than stating what you wish to not do. I'll show you an example of what I mean.

Let's say you have a sister who seems to have made a hobby of calling you and complaining about the way you treat her. Of course, you feel that you treat her perfectly fine, that you are loving and respectful toward her, and that you are always sensitive toward her and her feelings, but because she perceives things differently, these calls seem to come your way all the time...and, naturally, you always get upset when these phone calls conclude.

Now, most people, if they decided they no longer wanted to be upset after these phone calls, would make a statement such as this: "Next time she calls, I am not going to get upset." While that is a great resolution, however, you would be failing, in this example, to give yourself a *positive alternative*. In other words, it's not about what you are *not going to do*, but is instead about what you are *going to do*. Instead of saying, "Next time she calls, *I am not going* to get upset," it would be far more beneficial for you to say, "Next time she calls, *I am going* to go for a walk afterward and listen to that favorite song of mine that always calms me down." You see?

By providing yourself with a positive alternative, you will give yourself something you are going to do in order to solve the problem, rather than simply stating what you are not going to do. Because it is often external influences that can cause huge swings in our emotions; coming up with positive-minded solutions for recurring problems can be a great way to keep your emotions strong and balanced.

A major aspect of the state of our emotions is the negativity we are allowing into our lives, or the positivity we are pulling into our lives. And because our emotions not only have an impact on our health, but also have a major impact on whether we are truly "thriving" in life instead of just "surviving," it is important that you are consciously purposing to adhere to the principles of positive thinking.

3.   Get plenty of sleep

As much as I would love to prescribe a certain, specific number of hours of sleep to you that you "should get every night," the truth is that pretty much every different study on sleep seems to come up with a different "exact number of hours we are supposed to get." What I can tell you is that there are very few people who can get by with six or fewer hours of sleep while still enabling their body to recover and become properly rejuvenated each night. Of course, there are some of us who love sleep and do not need to be told twice that we should be getting plenty of sleep each night.

At the same time, any collection of people tends to have one or two stubborn individuals who claim to loathe the necessity of sleep, and who have attempted for years to get by on far fewer hours than their body actually needs.

If you fall into this second category, realize this: Although it may seem, for a while, as though you are doing just fine on fewer hours of sleep than you should be getting, this consistent lack of sleep will eventually catch up to your mind and body, and there is a very good chance it is already catching up to your emotions.

After all, sleep deprivation has been associated with high blood pressure, obesity, and diabetes. Sleep is also necessary to allow memories to stick, what the experts call "memory consolidation, as well as enabling you to absorb and recall new information.

An interesting MRI brain scan study at Harvard concerning sleep showed that while you sleep, you are shifting memories to more efficient storage areas within the brain[5]. How wild is that. Therefore, when you wake up, memory tasks can be performed more accurately, more quickly, and more effectively, with less anxiety and stress building up in your life, as your mind will be less cluttered.

Some experts have even theorized that this is why infants require so much sleep, as they are undertaking enormous amounts of learning, and therefore need the time to sleep at night in order to consolidate these memories and place them in areas of the brain where they will stick.

And when it comes to older people, a unique challenge arises in relation to sleep activity, as sleep quality deteriorates mostly in the form of a decrease in slow wave activity, which contributes to a decline in the ability to establish long-term memories. The older brain then relies more heavily on the area that is designated for short-term memory storage, and so,

---

[5] "Study Shows How Sleep Improves Memory", Beth Israel Deaconess Medical Center. Retrieved January 16, 2015 from http://www.sciencedaily.com/releases/2005/06/050629070337.htm

the brain has a tendency to become cluttered because the memories will not move into long-term storage as effectively as the younger brain.

In other words, a good night of sleep goes a long way, and one of the best ways to make sure you are getting a good night of sleep is by exercising sometime during the day (preferably not right before bedtime.), as this will go a long way toward ensuring your sleep is as deep and complete as it needs to be.

While the best general prescription regarding "the amount of sleep you should get" puts the average person at around eight hours per night, the real truth is that each human body is engineered slightly differently, and some people certainly do need more sleep than others.

As such, you should make a concerted effort to pay attention to how you feel with different durations of hours of sleep. If you are getting too little sleep, you will tend to feel tired all day, and if you are getting too much sleep, you may find that you are left feeling perpetually sluggish.

Once you find that middle ground, the place at which you feel refreshed and lively throughout the day, you will then want to aim to get that amount of sleep each and every night. This will go a long way toward keeping your body replenished and healthy, and will have a tangibly positive impact on your overall emotional state.

4.   Laugh.

There is a common saying regarding laughter that you have surely heard before: "Laughter is the best medicine." And while I would not go so far myself as to say laughter is the best medicine, there is certainly no disputing the fact that laughter can be immensely beneficial for your emotional state. And, of course, this translates to laughter being great for your physical body as well.

People who laugh have been found to have less of the stress hormone cortisol. A study at Vanderbilt University estimated that just 10 to 15 minutes of laughter can burn 40 calories, and the University of Maryland found that laughter can actually protect against heart disease. In fact, researchers go on to say that putting laughter into your daily routine through social interactions with friends, group exercise, or even watching humor on television will enhance your learning ability and improve your ability to recall. As such, I recommend plan a dose of laughter in anyone's wellness. It will improve your body, mind, and spirit.

What makes you laugh? Think about it. Is it a certain television show? A certain comedian? Time spent with a particular friend? Regardless of what it is that makes you laugh, realize that you should aim to engage with this source of laughter on a regular basis.

Life is just more fun when laughter is involved...and that, certainly, is a large part of *LIVING BETTER*. Learn to incorporate laughter into your day-to-day life, and positive results will follow.

5.   Find friends with whom you can enjoy life

Generally speaking, each of us has different friends who serve different purposes in our lives. Perhaps you have one friend who seemingly has you in their life simply so they can complain to you about everything going on in their own life. Or, perhaps you have a friend who only wants to talk about their own self.

Maybe you have friends you don't particularly care for, and maybe you have friends you feel like you hardly even know. It's great to have all sorts of friends who are in our lives for all sorts of different purposes, but there is truly nothing more special and wonderful than having friends with whom you can genuinely enjoy life. Human beings, after all, are social creatures.

We have all heard this before, but many of us fail to realize just how true this really is. The John Hopkins University School of Public Health recently found out that social isolation is associated with dementia. Spending time with others was better than crossword puzzles in middle-age and later life in preventing memory loss and improving overall physical health.

Research from Stockholm, Sweden has suggested that we could get much more "bang for our buck" when we combine activities that include mental or physical exercise along with social interaction. Some great examples of this may be joining a bowling league, playing bridge, chess, or a game of cards, or simply riding a bike with a group of friends. In the same study, it stated that dancing is the best activity of all, as it involves both physical and social interaction.

Think about your group of friends, and identify the individuals around whom you have the most fun, the individuals with whom you can most fully enjoy life. If you are able to identify a handful of friends in your life who fit this description, realize that it will be worth it for you to make an effort to spend time around these friends as often as you can.

And if you are unable to identify any friends of yours whom you would label as being "friends with whom I can enjoy life," it's time to start meeting some new friends, friends who can fulfill this purpose for you... friends, also, for whom you can fulfill this purpose as well.

6.   Have fun.

Fill in the blank. "Life is _____." All the time, I hear people say things like, "Life is hard," or "Life is difficult," or "Life is a trial." But if you can get rid of such negative thoughts, you will come to realize what life really is, what life really can be for those who so desire, is fun.

That's right, life is fun! Sure, you might have problems. Hey, we all do. Sure, things may be difficult at times, and life may not always go the way you planned it. But when it comes down to it, life is an adventure, a spontaneous adventure.

And when you begin to look at life through this lens, you will soon discover that life is in fact fun. You will soon discover that life is a marvelous gift, and you will become far more intentional about *LIVING LONGER AND BETTER* so you can enjoy this wonderful life for as long as possible.

One of the most important things to realize with regards to the idea of life being truly "fun" is the fact that things in life will not always go perfectly. But even when things do not go perfectly, life can still be perfectly fun. After all, part of the adventure inherent in life is the unpredictability and the spontaneity of it all.

Once you start looking at life through the lens of it being a truly fun, rewarding, adventurous experience, you will begin to discover that all of this is true. Life is fun. And as you have fun making your way through this adventure of life, your emotions will be lifted, and your physical health will be lifted, and *LIVING LONGER AND BETTER* will suddenly become a far more attainable goal.

7. Be *INTENTIONAL* with your emotions

Because the very nature of emotions, as mentioned at the beginning of this section, is abstractness... because, that is to say, emotions have no physical form outside of the names we ascribe to various emotions, it is sometimes difficult for us to give emotions the proper amount of thought and attention they deserve.

In order to ensure that your emotions are properly balanced, and in order to get the greatest positive impact from your emotional state, you will need to spend some time focusing on your emotions in a conscious, intentional manner.

Start taking the time to identify certain emotions you have in certain situations, and assess the manner in which these emotions are affecting your physical and mental state. Identify the sources of negative emotions, and come up with "action plans" you can implement in order to combat these negative emotions when they come upon you.

And, of course, identify the sources of positive emotions, and make sure you are indulging in the roots of these positive emotions as often as you can. It may seem like a small thing, but in the long run, having a balanced and positive emotional state can make a massive difference.

"An action plan? What, exactly, does this look like?" Simply stated, an action plan is a technique to overcome negative emotions. Negative emotions will get in your way of living longer and better, and one of the most effective ways to turn negative emotions and stress into something positive is by doing the following: Say to yourself, "I am going to write down 10 things that I feel happy about in my life."

Alternately, another group of people may say, "I am going to write down 10 things I am grateful to God for," and another group may say, "I am going to intentionally change all my negative thoughts into positive ones." As I discussed earlier, this was my tactic when I was dealing with thinning hair, and trust me when I say, this really works.

Furthermore, think back to our example of the sister calling and having the hobby of complaining about the way she is treated. What is your action plan here? You could choose to open up to her and tell her your true feelings rather than holding them inside.

Some people may experience barriers that seem insurmountable, but there are techniques to succeed. If the barrier that you are facing seems so bad you cannot think of any positive, simply wait for a moment when you are feeling good, and make a list of the positive things, then save it for when you feel down.

Truly, these things will make a major difference in your quality of life, and will have a huge impact on the level of positivity in your emotional state.

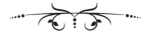

7 Keys to a *LIVING LONGER AND BETTER:*

<u>Spirituality</u>

1. Spend time in silence

Of course, you have heard it said before that "silence is golden." This may seem like an overstatement, or like something akin to pure hyperbole, but honestly, this statement is closer to truth than you may have ever thought.

While many of us would state, without much reservation, that we certainly get a bit of silence in our lives, most of us are nevertheless astonished when we find ourselves in a true place of stillness and silence. Not only are we astonished to discover that this is, in fact, something we are not at all used to, but we are also astonished to discover just how rejuvenating and replenishing a bit of true "stillness and silence" can be.

Even if you are not a religious person yourself, or are not particularly interested in spirituality as a whole, you will certainly come to realize, and will certainly agree with my assertion, that there is something truly special and rewarding about a bit of time spent in this state.

One of the most important things to realize, if you are wanting to reach a place from which you will be able to enjoy the rejuvenating effects of true stillness and silence, is that it is often difficult to really reach a place of stillness and silence in your familiar surroundings and your everyday life.

Of course, once you become accustomed to really indulging in stillness and silence from time to time, it will become easier for you to slip into this restful place for a few minutes at a time, even within the hustle and bustle of your daily life. But until you reach that place yourself, you will need to make a concerted effort to truly provide yourself with opportunities to replenish yourself. If you are comfortable with outdoor activities, going camping for a night (or even two) can be an excellent way to enjoy the sort of stillness and organic silence that is so difficult for us to achieve in our daily lives. But there are also plenty of other options for reaching this place if camping is something that does not appeal to you.

For instance, you could take a canoe out to the middle of a lake and just simply rest there for a while, or you could rent a cabin in a place with no cell phone service or internet connection and unwind for a day, or , if you have the discipline to do so, you could even create your own "cabin with no cell phone service or internet connection" right in your own home by simply putting your phone on airplane mode and turning off your computer (and your television) for a day, using this day to rest and relax with no external noise bombarding you, and with nothing to keep you busy and stimulated other than your own thoughts and the silence around you.

And let me tell you, if this sounds difficult or challenging to you, then there is a good chance this is exactly what you need. As you learn to enjoy and thrive in silence, you will create opportunities for silence to work its magic on your, and to positively impact your life. This will ultimately lead you to a place where your capacity for *LIVING LONGER AND BETTER* is significantly increased.

2. Spend time connecting with something greater

For myself, "connecting with something greater" means spending time in prayer, spending time reading my Bible, attending church on Sundays, and discussing areas of faith with my wife and family.

For others, "connecting with something greater" can mean meditation, or can mean prayer and reading which can be focused on another form of religion. Once more, even if you are not religious, and even if you are not particularly "into spirituality," the idea of "connecting with something greater" than yourself is still an important aspect to pay attention to.

As counterintuitive as it may sound on the surface, you will discover that, once you reach a point from which you are able to connect with something greater than yourself and, as a result, are able to let go of your compulsion to try to control and "be in charge" of every area of your life, you will achieve a much higher level of peace, and a much greater feeling of safety and security.

By letting go of the amount of control you are attempting to exert in your own life, the more peaceful and at ease you are going to feel. And this is what "connecting with something greater" enables you to do.

As mentioned already, "connecting with something greater," for me, means prayer, Bible reading, church attendance, and discussions of faith. If you adhere to beliefs in another area of religion, you probably know exactly what enables you to connect with something greater than yourself (not to say that you always make the appropriate amount of effort to actually connect in the way you would like. Hey, it is something we all have difficulties doing at one time or another of our lives.) At least you know what these "things that enable you to connect to something greater" are, and are able to then make a concerted effort to connect as fully as you can in these ways. But if you are not into spirituality yourself and are not a particularly religious person, it may be difficult to determine what this "something greater than yourself" is.

While it is certainly true that different things can work for different people, most people in this position discover that making an effort to achieve a close connection with the Earth itself is a great way to "connect with something greater."

By spending time outdoors and really making a strong effort to enjoy nature, you will also create a corresponding "spiritual peace" (or even "spiritual enlightenment"), a sort of epiphany, that is to say, that goes something like this:

"Why do I spend time and energy worrying about the little things in my life that are ultimately so unimportant, when the world is so much bigger than me? After all, I can only control the things that I can control, and the rest will ultimately take care of itself." This will end up leading to a much greater sense of peace, and will help you enjoy each day as it comes.

Even if spending time outdoors and enjoying nature are not ideas that sound particularly appealing to you, this is nevertheless something that will be immensely beneficial for you when you take steps toward doing it.

Furthermore, spending time outdoors and enjoying nature can be great ways for you to make sure you are taking care of your physical fitness, remaining healthy in your body, while simultaneously enhancing your spirituality...each of which will go a long way toward helping you *LIVE LONGER AND BETTER.*

Finally, realize that nature and connecting with the Earth are not the only options available to those of you who are not particularly religiously-inclined (and what's more, nature and connecting with the Earth are not exclusive to those who are not religiously-inclined; even if you are a religious person, enjoying nature and connecting with the Earth can contribute greatly to your spiritual enhancement and inner peace).

Other options for "connecting to something greater" include immersing yourself in the animal kingdom, spending time on the open ocean, and purchasing a telescope that you can use for looking into the cosmos. Those are just a few of the many ways in which you can effectively connect with something greater than yourself.

3.   Eliminate hectic areas of your life

One of the most effective ways to destroy your spiritual enhancement and your sense of inner peace is by getting too caught up in the areas of your life that cause you to feel hectic and frenetic.

If you start to feel as though the pieces of your life are comparable to a bag of bouncing balls that has been opened and poured onto a wooden floor, with these bouncing balls rolling and bouncing every which way and foiling your desperate attempts to recapture them all, this is probably an indication that you need to pause. Take a breath. Pull your focus back into a deeper, more "centered" place.

When we get too caught up in the little things, trying to control all these little things and corral them together, we doom ourselves to ending up in a place from which we are achieving less inner peace and spiritual enhancement than is optimal.

When it comes down to it, none of us will be able to ever control all those little things in our lives; by their very nature, most of these little things that cause us to feel so thinly-spread are outside of our control to begin with, and all we accomplish by trying to corral and control these things is this: We end up feeling significantly more stressed and unsettled than we should, for absolutely no reason whatsoever.

A large part of the "help for reaching a place from which we are no longer trying to control all the little things in our life" will come from our ability to successfully connect with "something greater."

Victor Frank (famous psychiatrist and holocaust survivor) once wrote: "He who has the why can bear anyhow." I believe, in writing this, he was pointing out that when we reach beyond ourselves and connect to something greater, we begin to answer the "why" for the reasons we are trying to achieve a certain goal.

Andrew Shatte stated it nicely when he said, "At the basic level, we have individual goals," something that we would like to achieve, whether it's money, a certain standard of living, or simple pleasure and satisfaction[6]. When we take it a step further and connect our ambitions to something greater, like our family or our community or even God or something spiritual, this thing we have a desire to achieve will outlast or outlive us.

As we begin to connect to something greater than ourselves, our level of satisfaction and resilience will automatically increase, because we are doing something that goes beyond ourselves. When you begin to connect on a deeper level with something greater than yourself, these little things, these hectic things that we try so hard to control, in spite of our inability to ever truly control them, will finally be revealed to you to be exactly what they are; little things.

Even still, however, actively aiming to connect with something greater is not going to be enough on its own to lead you to a place from which you can truly let

---

[6] Reivich, K. & Shatte, A. "The Resilience Factor: 7 Essential Skills for Overcoming Life's Inevitable Obstacles." Retrieved September 3, 2015 from http://www.davidsongifted.org/db/Articles_id_10552.aspx

go of all these hectic areas of your life. In order to truly reach that point, you will also need to be *intentional* in your efforts to do so.

As you move through life, aim to identify the "little things" that end up causing you to feel as though life is far more hectic than it should be. And then, as you manage to actively identify these little things, it will become far easier for you to actively and *intentionally* eliminate your compulsion to corral and control all these little things you will be unable to corral and control anyway. This will leave you with far fewer things to worry about in life, and will make life a lot more pleasant and spiritually rewarding as a result.

I have also found that learning how to say "No" can be extremely liberating when you first experience it, and can go a long way toward eliminating stress. Recently, I was supposed to be at a certain place to discuss the care of an individual; it was something extra I had been asked to do, but nevertheless, I had agreed to it.

The day came when I was supposed to be there, and wouldn't you know it, five other, more important things hit me all at the same time. On that day, I had to make a decision; I had to prioritize my time (an everyday occurrence for most physicians, but on this particular day, it was more of a challenge, because I had made a commitment to a friend).

After assessing things realistically, however, I had to say "No" to the friend, and you know what? The following day, the family called and all but apologized, saying they understood how busy my schedule is, and we were then able to handle everything over the phone.

I felt completely liberated when I was able to make a choice, when I was able to prioritize and, ultimately, say "No, I cannot be there." This little lesson was very instructive to me, and I think it will help you too. Saying "No" is an excellent way to reduce stress.

Another way I learned to reduce stress and make things less hectic in my life is by making time for myself. For example: three days a week, I end office hours at 3:30 and commit that time to exercise.

No matter what happens earlier in the day, I have my private exercise time to look forward to; no meetings, no appointments, and the emergency room will handle any unexpected illnesses. It is easy to get super stressed with the hectic day of a physician, but as long as I know I can either bike, run, swim, or lift weight (or any combination of the above), I feel invincible in my mind as I move through the day.

This single aspect of my life has worked miracles, as that time when I am running, swimming, or on my bike is a time when I am completely disconnected from and out of touch with the professional world.

4. Think long-term

One of the big things that causes many of us to fail in our efforts to achieve a high level of inner peace and spiritual enlightenment is that we are far more short-term-focused than we should be.

When we are focused on the short-term areas of our lives, we ultimately end up experiencing far more highs and lows in our day-to-day lives than we should. Every small thing that goes well in our life causes us to enjoy a big, upward swing...which is all good and well, until the next small thing that goes poorly in our life causes us to dip far lower than anyone has any desire to dip. This creates a sort of roller coaster in our lives, what I like to refer to, in fact, as a "blindfolded roller coaster," where you are not only experiencing extreme highs and lows on a daily basis, but are also blind to what will be coming next.

Will we experience the joy of another high point today? Or will we instead be stuck facing the devastation of another extreme low? This is detrimental to our spiritual, emotional, and mental states, which not only means that we enjoy life less as a result, but also means that our physical state is negatively affected, thereby putting us in a worsened position for enjoying a long, healthy life...negatively affecting, that is to say, our ability to *LIVE LONGER AND BETTER.*

"But, Dr. Andrew, I'm 80 years old. You want me to 'think long-term'?"

Absolutely. No matter your age, your outlook on life should always be something like this: "I want to live life in the moment, enjoying the gift of each day without worrying about all the little things that make my life seem more hectic than it really is, and as I live life in the moment and enjoy the gift of each day, I want to also purpose to keep my eyes on my long-term goals and on the big picture of my life and future." Yes. Future.

Because as long as you are still alive and breathing, you have a future ahead of you. Too many of us get tied up by our ideas of how long life is going to be, or, worse, of how long we will be able to lead a healthy, rewarding life. As we predict, in our minds (and sometimes even aloud), that we only have until the age of 75, or only have until the age of 80, or only have until the age of 90, before we will die, or before we will physically and mentally disintegrate, we ultimately end up directing our body to make that proclamation a reality.

On the other hand, when we keep our eyes toward the future, living with long-term goals and the big-picture at the forefront of our minds, we ultimately direct our bodies to keep us going, and to put us in a position to reach those goals and desires we have set before us.

As a side note; if you think you "only have until the age of 75," or "only have until the age of 80," or "only have until the age of 90," it's about time you start paying attention to all the individuals out there who have led healthy, rewarding lives to the age of 100, and even, in many cases, beyond. Stay long-term focused, and you will be able to direct your body to accomplish this as well.

5. Actively monitor your inner peace

Many times in this section, we have mentioned "inner peace." One thing to realize, however, is that your inner peace is not going to reach a high level by accident; instead, you need to actively monitor your inner peace, and need to gauge your level of inner peace on a daily basis.

On days when you gauge your inner peace and can honestly say, "Hey, how about that, I feel really peaceful today," it will then be worthwhile to assess your present situation and determine what has led to you feeling calm and peaceful on this particular day.

And if you gauge your inner peace and say, "Hmmm, I am feeling very unsettled, very 'unpeaceful', today," you will want to then take a look at your life and determine what is causing you to feel unsettled in that moment.

The more active you are in your efforts to monitor your inner peace, the more practice you will attain with regards to identifying both positives and negatives in your life that have an impact on your inner peace.

And as you gain more clarity on the elements in your life that cause your inner peace to improve, and on elements in your life that cause your inner peace to dwindle, you will find that you are in a better position to regularly (and subconsciously) keep your inner peace at a high level, and will be able to enjoy a far more rewarding, fruitful, and beneficial existence as a result.

6. Find ways to help others.

One of the big areas in which most people fail in life is the fact that their perspective on life reaches only as far as their own self, their own triumphs, their own disappointments, and their own experiences.

In fact, this is the natural inclination most human beings have; think of "self" first, and worry about others if time and energy permit. What you will find, however, if you instead take the time and make a concerted effort to place a heavy focus in your life on "others," is that life becomes significantly more enjoyable and rewarding when you are doing what you can to make the world a better place for others.

The world, after all, is much greater (and much broader) than your own experiences, your own dreams, your own triumphs, your own fears, and your own disappointments.

The world is a finely-woven tapestry, encompassing all individuals, all across the world, in all walks of life.

When you tie yourself into this tapestry more fully and completely, this will not only provide you with another way of connecting with something greater, but will also create a greater level of purpose and accomplishment within yourself (leading, of course, to an increased inner peace). The more you help others, the more you ultimately end up helping yourself.

While you may not have thought of it before, it is worth noting that there are actually plenty of opportunities for seniors to serve in their communities. For example, did you know that one of the best ways to contribute, as a senior, is by donating time to other seniors?

Individuals in nursing homes, for example, always come away feeling refreshed and replenished when they are able to spend time around healthy seniors, and seniors who are stuck spending plenty of their time in the hospital tend to show improvement after a healthy dose of visits from healthy friends and family members.

Even if you do not have any close friends who are dealing with health issues, and even if there is not a nursing home in your area at which you can volunteer, simply doing little things to make life easier for your peers can be a great way to boost the lives of these individuals, and to boost your own life as a result.

And, of course, there are always plenty of opportunities for "helping others" outside of simply helping seniors. Regardless of whether you choose to volunteer at a soup kitchen or choose to provide services to underprivileged families, you will discover that you enjoy a greater sense of purpose when you are taking the time to help others.

And you will also find that it becomes far easier to let go of the "little problems" (the little problems we talked about earlier that can be so difficult, at times, to let go of.) when you begin to see (and help with) the far bigger problems others in the world are dealing with.

This will lead to a greatly-enhanced sense of inner peace and spiritual strength, which will lead to a healthier mental and emotional state, and will ultimately lead to a healthier body...making it far easier for you to LIVE LONGER AND BETTER.

7.   Be *INTENTIONAL* with the spiritual side of your life

As with physical fitness, mental sharpness, and emotional stability, spiritual enhancement does not occur by accident. In order to enjoy the benefits of a strong spiritual side to your life, you are going to need to be *intentional* in your efforts to make this happen.

You will need to closely monitor your spirituality; you will need to keep close tabs on your inner peace; you will need to pay attention to the things you can and should be doing in order to connect to "something greater than yourself" and increase your inner peace; you will need to be *intentional*.

It may take a bit of time to reach this place, but when you are intentional with your spirituality, this will lead to a far more rewarding life, and will make it significantly easier for you to truly live a life that is long, healthy, and consistently enjoyable.

THE MISHANDLING OF MODERN MEDICINE

Medicine can be tremendously beneficial. But mishandled medicine can wreck an older individual's shot at a long, healthy life.

Okay, now that the title of this chapter caught your attention...

Seriously, though, I want to start out this chapter by saying that I have absolutely nothing against medicine. I use medicine myself, and I certainly prescribe medicine to my patients. Modern medicine is an amazing thing, and the amount of progress we have made over the years in eradicating certain diseases and battling other diseases is astonishing, all of it attributable to the incredible power and progress of modern medicine.

Furthermore, medicine can be an incredibly effective "helper" for individuals in their older years. Certain medicines can help to turn the tide of troublesome illnesses and diseases; other medicines can help to eradicate pain in places where nothing else will do. Without modern medicine, our ability to even reach those older years, let alone our ability to enjoy those older years, would be much weaker, and I certainly do not want to take away from that.

At the same time, however, there is a point at which modern medicine becomes a crutch. There is a point at which doctors find themselves prescribing medicine in order to simply cover up the proverbial fruit of a problem, when they should instead be looking for ways in which to take care of the root of that problem. There is a point at which medicine even becomes an obstacle in the way of great health, instead of aiding our pursuit of a world in which each of us is equipped to *LIVE LONGER AND BETTER*.

In order for medicine to truly do what it is intended to do, we must find the balance between medicine and natural healing.

Let's talk a bit about overmedication. This is, by no means, a thorough exploration of the overmedication problem, but I do want to give you a few examples of what this looks like, in order to give you an idea of the sorts of things patients deal with without even realizing it.

One of the big issues with geriatric care is that arteries get stiff, which is why I advise all patients to have a blood pressure machine at home. Many patients, when sitting in a medical office and surrounded by this uncomfortable setting, end up dealing with "white coat hypertension," which causes their blood pressure to shoot up to 200 when the doctor is testing it, when in reality this patient's blood pressure is 130 when they are relaxed in the comfort of their own home.

Because the doctor is unable to get an accurate reading on the patient's blood pressure, they prescribe medication that does not need to be prescribed in the first place, and the patient ends up getting dizzy and light-headed; the patient ends up falling at home, because of this overmedication.

A further example of overmedication that stands out to me was a few years ago when the Joint and National Committee on Blood Pressure said that the first line of treatment should be a diuretic, HCTZ.

At the time, I told my brother-in-law that the guy on the committee obviously did not practice medicine, as HCTZ was the worst thing you could give an older patient, as it would lower their blood sodium, leading them to become confused, to fall over, to break a hip, etc.

Sure enough, when the J&C 8 met five years later, they decided that HCTZ was dangerous for older people. This was after five years of them encouraging doctors to prescribe HCTZ as a first line of defense against higher blood pressure.

We could also look at diabetes, another one of the major problem areas for overmedication. As anyone with diabetes knows, we have a glycol hemoglobin that tells us how our blood sugar has been over the last six weeks, which gives us a measure of how bad the diabetes is.

The higher the blood sugar, the higher the glycol hemoglobin (the "A1c"). When we are dealing with this in older people, I have found that they need an A1c of eight, which means, essentially, that they can tolerate a higher blood sugar level, but the chances of hypoglycemia are much less.

Consistently, however, I see patients going to the emergency room because their blood sugar is low... because the doctor they were going to told them they should have an A1c of six. An A1c of six is how I treat my 50-year-olds, but an 80-year-old should not be treated the same way as a 50-year-old.

Antidepressants being prescribed to older individuals is another major area of overmedication, or really, frankly, of misdiagnosis. Most primary care doctors are not trained to deal with depression or over-depression in older individuals, as depression in older individuals is manifested quite differently from depression in a younger patient.

Many older patients deal with a type of depression that is manifested with a large component of anxiety. We commonly refer to this as "anxious depression," and it represents up to 75% of all older age depression. The average primary care doctor will prescribe a drug such as Prozac when depression is so much as mentioned, regardless of whether the patient is old or young, but because of the nature of Prozac, it tends to make anxiety worse.

Why would anyone want to give an individual who is dealing with anxious depression a medication that will make them more anxious? Furthermore, Prozac can cause a decrease in appetite, which can cause an older patient to lose weight. Are there older patients who do benefit from drugs such as Prozac and Wellbutrin?

Of course, there are still 25% of older individuals whose depression is not categorized as anxious depression. But without a proper examination and diagnosis, many older patients are being led astray.

And to give you an idea of exactly what the over medication problem can look like... one of the worst areas of all is depressive medications. Although most primary care doctors are not particularly trained or equipped to deal with depression (and because there are not many geriatric psychiatrists out there), many primary care doctors will prescribe medications such as Prozac or Effexor, which are contra-indicative in older people, as these medicines are activating.

Of course, these medicines can work quite well for younger people who do not feel like getting out of bed or do not feel like doing anything at all, as these medicines can push them to become more active. For unmotivated older people, however, something needs to be prescribed that will take the edge off their anxiety and increase their mood, which calls for medication that takes care of anxious depression, such as Celexa or Citalopram.

And in the meantime, the doctor should be working to take care of the root of the problem, i.e., what is causing the depression, rather than simply prescribing medication that will mask the problem.

There is so much misinformation out there regarding the medication of older patients, and this leads to a great number of patients taking more medicine than they should, and, even worse, taking the wrong medicines...medicines that are exacerbating the problems (or are creating new problems) rather than contributing to a solution.

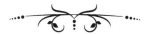

As doctors, we are here to help others live better lives. When it comes down to it, this is what our profession is really all about. After all, "health" is a huge part of living a life that is as pleasant and fulfilling as it should be, and our entire job is predicated upon a search for the ways in which your health can be improved.

This, however, is where a lot of the issues end up coming into play, in regards to overmedication. After all, not all problems can be gotten rid of, or, more accurately, not all problems can be gotten rid of easily, as there are certainly problems that cannot be gotten rid of.

But these are problems we run into far less often than those problems that are difficult to get rid of. As doctors, then, we want to find a way to "make things better," to "help others live better lives" right away, and this is why so many doctors prescribe medicine to "ease discomfort," even if these medicines sometimes do nothing to help solve the problem...even if these medicines, in fact, sometimes end up further contributing to the problems.

The way I like to illustrate this is in the following manner:

Think of a tree that has bugs eating its roots. As the bugs continue to chip away at the roots, there are going to branches on the tree itself (on the visible portion of the tree, that is) that end up dying. This is the sign we see from the outside, the dead branches on the visible portion of the tree. As such, there are two solutions we could come up with.

Firstly, we could trim the dead branches, in order to ensure that the tree continues to look good on the outside...until; eventually the work of those bugs goes so far that the tree finally dies. Or, we could instead take steps to eradicate the bugs themselves. This would take more work, of course, but by getting rid of the bugs, we would get rid of the problem altogether.

This is very similar to the way modern medicine is often handled. Instead of finding medicine that works to kill the "bugs," medicine is prescribed to "trim the branches," to make things look okay on the outside, covering up the symptoms of what is really ailing the patient.

Of course, even as you take steps to kill the bugs in the example above, you could still continue to trim branches as well, ensuring that the tree looks good on the outside, as you solve the problems going on beneath the surface, and the same can certainly be done with modern medicine. It is perfectly fine to take medicine that "trims the branches," that takes care of the symptoms, that is, but we should still be striving to figure out the root of the problem at the same time.

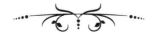

What is really sad, however, is that so many retired individuals have bought into the idea that this is "how things are supposed to go." They go along with this method of "fixing the symptoms," and they do this largely because they assume they can trust their doctor to make the best decisions for them (after all, if they cannot trust their doctor with their health, who can they trust?).

Furthermore, this is not to imply that doctors are doing this maliciously or negligently. It is not as though doctors are examining patients and saying, "Well, sure, we could do a lot more work and try to solve the problem, but let's just make things easier on ourselves by simply covering up the symptoms." Not at all.

Instead, the issue is simply that most doctors do not recognize the ways in which these problems can be solved...most doctors do not understand that solving these problems at their root will often require them to go beyond medicine.

In the same way most people in their 60s, 70s, 80s, and 90s have bought into the idea that there is really very little for us to do beyond "surviving" as the years advance, many doctors have bought into this idea as well. This leads them to look for ways to ease the state of "survival," to "make patients comfortable" and fix the symptoms of the problems patients are dealing with, rather than looking for ways to help patients truly become better.

After all, if a doctor fails to recognize just how "exceptional" it is possible for the years after retirement to be, and when a large part of the elements that will contribute to someone being an "exceptional retired individual" come from areas that are not strictly within the bounds of modern medicine, how can you then expect them to truly take the right steps to ensure someone is leading a complete and optimal retired life.

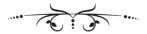

Is medicine good? Yes, absolutely. However, in-and-of-itself, medicine is not enough, and this is especially true when medicine is used simply to improve the state of someone's survival, rather than being used to help someone's quest to thrive.

It is time for the medical community to progress beyond the point where we are simply content with medicine masking the problems. Instead, we need to reach a point where we are working to eradicate the problems themselves.

And while this is something I will continue to push the medical community toward, doing everything I can do myself to help other doctors understand exactly what we ought to be doing in order to help patients truly get the most out of life, it will also be important for you, as an individual, to start understanding the role modern medicine plays in the minds of most doctors.

If you are being prescribed medicine, do not be afraid to ask questions. Be willing to ask the doctor exactly what your problem is (not the "fruit" of the problem, but instead, the "root" of the problem). Then ask them for details on exactly how the medicine is helping to take care of and eradicate the problem.

It is not hyperbole; truly, honestly, and genuinely, each of us has the capacity to LIVE LONGER AND BETTER, and to enjoy exceptional health and an extraordinary life deep into our 70s, 80s, and 90s.

Once you grasp the concept of taking care of your whole "self," of looking after not only your body, but also your mind, your emotions, and your spirituality, and once you combine this with a full-fledged belief that it is possible for you to lead a strong, healthy life, you will put yourself in position to truly count yourself amongst the "exceptional retired individuals."

"THE NOT-SO-PERFECT LIFE"?

Let's place you inside the life that far too many retired individuals lead. This life could easily be classified as "not so perfect."

It does not matter what month it is, or even what day of the week it is, because every month, and every day, is pretty much the same to you. After all, what does it matter what the weather is like outside, when you really do not ever leave the house?

And what does it matter what day of the week it is? It's all arbitrary anyway, right? Just a way for the working world to stay on a cohesive schedule. For you, the retired individual, it may as well be a Saturday in June as a Monday in January. As long as it is not a holiday, it makes very little difference to you.

You stay in bed for a bit upon waking up, as you do not particularly feel like getting up just yet. Perhaps you even toss and turn for a bit, trying to get back to sleep, but eventually you acknowledge that a return to sleep is not in the cards, so you swing your feet onto the floor and shuffle to the kitchen.

You prepare your coffee and make a bowl of oatmeal, and your morning routine is complete. You now shuffle to the living room and sit down in your recliner and flip on the television. For the next few hours, you flip through different morning shows. For the most part, commercial spots line up across the different channels, so this means you also spend about 20% of your morning watching commercials, mostly for cleaning products, and for other items marketed toward seniors and stay-at-home moms.

Around noon, you realize you never opened the curtains in the living room. The only source of light is the television itself. You consider getting up from the recliner to open the curtains and at least see what the day looks like...but then, you really do not feel like getting up at the moment.

In fact, you are quite tired. You pick up the remote control and mute the television, and you close your eyes and nap in your chair for an hour or two.

When you wake up, you have to go to the bathroom. You stand up and shuffle to the bathroom, and you figure that while you are up, you may as well make lunch, that way, you won't have to get up again just for that. You head to the kitchen and make a sandwich, and you bring this sandwich and a glass of water back to your recliner. You sit down once more, take the television off mute, and flip through the channels until you find something that catches your eye.

A few hours later, you get up to use the bathroom again, and you grab a snack from the kitchen for dinner, then you return to your recliner once more, where you remain for the last few hours of the day.

Finally, you shuffle back to the bedroom, and you climb into bed and sleep until morning...when you wake up once more and start all over again.

"THE PERFECT LIFE"?

Let's place you inside the life of what I like to call "the exceptional retired individual." This is the life of someone who is not only ensuring that they are in position to "live longer," but is also making the effort to "live better" along the way.

It's January, but you wouldn't know it from the weather outside your window. After all, you slept with the windows open, and you woke up to the sounds of the ocean and a warm, pleasant breeze trickling into the room. You swing your legs out of bed right away, excited for the day that lies before you.

You take a shower and put on your bathing suit. Then you sit on your balcony and enjoy breakfast along with the sound of the ocean and the warm breeze before heading down to the beach.

You spend the day relaxing on the beach, sipping cold drinks, and reading a good book. Occasionally, you even walk down to the water and wade out into the waves, allowing the movement and the pleasant scent of warm saltwater refresh you and awaken your senses.

At night, you eat at a restaurant on the beach that has great food and live music. You watch couples get up from their tables and dance with one another.

Afterward, you climb into bed and close your eyes with the sounds of the ocean serenading you into sleep.

It's February, but more importantly, it's the first Friday of the month, and that means it is game night with three of your closest friends. Tonight, you are the one in charge of hosting game night, so you inspect the house and make sure there is nothing that needs to be cleaned, nothing you have overlooked in your standard, weekly cleaning of the house.

Everything looks good, so you head to the kitchen and make the dinner you will be providing tonight.

After trying to think of something light yet tasty that you can prepare for dessert (and coming up with nothing), you head to the store to pick up some cookies. While you are out, you decide to stop at a coffee shop and read. For about a half hour, you sip your drink and enjoy your book, but eventually you set your book aside and decide to watch the people who bustle in and out of the coffee shop.

Finally, you head home, and you hop on the computer to check up on the day's news and on the Facebook statuses of family and friends before your "game night friends" arrive.

The four of you stay up later than any of you had intended, eating dinner, playing games, enjoying those cookies, and eventually setting aside the games and simply chatting and catching up. Then you say goodbye to your friends, get ready for bed, and fall into a deep, rewarding sleep.

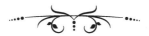

It's March, and you head out of the house almost the moment you wake up, as you have a breakfast date with a friend. The weather is surprisingly pleasant today, so the two of you decide to sit on the patio at the restaurant in order to take advantage of the fresh air.

The two of you have a great morning chatting, laughing, and catching up with one another, and then you hop in your car and drive to the gym. You do not particularly feel like doing anything too strenuous today, but you change into your bathing suit and take advantage of the gym's indoor pool, swimming a few laps to get your blood pumping and to get your muscles doing some work.

After taking a quick shower, you head home and decide to return to bed for a short nap. Upon waking up, you check to see if the weather is still pleasant (it is), then you put on your walking shoes and take a stroll through your neighborhood.

That night, you make dinner and enjoy a relaxing meal at home, then you head out to see a movie in theaters (with your significant other, or with a friend you have not seen in a while).

It's April, and it is a day you have had circled on your calendar for several weeks, as you and a group of friends are taking a drive to a nearby mountain, and are going to hike the trail that leads to the top (no, none of you expect to actually reach the top, but you are all excited to push yourselves and see how far up the mountain you can make it before it is time to turn around).

You wake up before the sun rises and put on the appropriate attire. Then you locate the backpack you purchased for this day; the backpack that has the water pouch inside it, and you fill the water pouch and toss a bag of trail mix and a few protein bars into the backpack as well. You shovel down a quick, protein-rich breakfast, and then you drive to meet your friends.

The drive to the mountain is worth the trip alone, as you and your friends spend the morning chatting, laughing, and making memories together. Finally, you reach the mountain itself, and, without over-thinking things (or pondering how sore all of you will probably be tomorrow), you start the hike.

It's not easy, but it is incredibly rewarding, as all of you push each other and encourage one another to keep making your way up the mountain. The path is well kept and not too steep, but the constant uphill movement and the thinning air notify you that this is more than just a normal walk.

Even still, by the time you turn around (more than a quarter of the way up the mountain, according to the markers on the path), all of you feel extremely proud and rejuvenated. The walk back down is easier, and the drive home is fairly quick. You crash that night the moment you arrive home, feeling extraordinarily exhausted, but also feeling as though the effort made and the task accomplished were very much worth it.

After all, it's not every day you get to go out and climb a mountain; it is a day worth being proud of, and it is a day you will remember for a long time to come.

It's May, and after a relaxing morning of breakfast, a book, a few puzzle games on the computer, and a bit of time sitting outside and enjoying the pleasant spring air, you get dressed for the afternoon.

Today, you and your significant other are going on a date that you have planned: the two of you will be driving out to a dude ranch, where a guide will take you on a horseback ride through the countryside. It's a scary thought, spending the day on the back of such a large animal, but it is thrilling as well, and as you and your significant other enjoy the fresh air and the open surroundings throughout the afternoon, you realize that you feel more closely-connected to the core of life than you have probably felt in ages.

That night, you pick up a carryout on your way home and sit in your most comfortable chair (which feels even more comfortable after sitting on a horse for hours that afternoon). Then you and your significant other pop in a favorite movie while you eat, rest, and recuperate from the day.

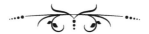

It's June, and you wake up and shower and then prepare breakfast. You decide to step outside to see what the weather is like today, and upon discovering that it is a perfect summer day (with that sultry summer air, but with temperatures that are not too hot for comfort), you decide to eat outside.

You finish eating and go back inside to clean your plate, and an idea hits you: Why stay inside all day when the air outside is so pleasant? Why not, instead, turn this into a classic summer day.

You open the refrigerator to see if you, by chance, have any lemonade in there. Nope, no lemonade. You ponder for a second whether or not it is worth a trip to the store for this, and finally you determine that a "classic summer day" just won't feel right unless you have some cold lemonade to go with it.

You drive to the store, pick up some lemonade, and come back home, and then you spend the rest of the day (one of the most pleasant and relaxing days you can remember having enjoyed in ages) sitting on the patio with a book and a regularly replenished glass of ice-cold lemonade.

As the day winds down, you decide that, sure, you did not exactly do anything long-lasting or "rewarding" with your day, but you nevertheless enjoyed the day immensely, and you would do it again in a heartbeat. Truly, it was the sort of day life is made for; a day of complete relaxation and absolute enjoyment.

It's July, and as you eat breakfast and think about what you want to do with the day, you start thinking about the places of your surrounding areas that you have never visited or properly explored before. You hop online and start to research some of the towns around you, and you discover that one of the towns in your area is renowned for its antique shops. How about that?

You throw on some clothes that will be suitable for walking, and you ask your significant other or a close friend if they want to join you today as you explore a new town.

The two of you drive to this town and pass the afternoon ducking in and out of antique shops and wandering the streets of this cute little town. You actually end up purchasing nothing throughout the day, but it is nevertheless extremely pleasant and rewarding to simply peruse these shops and see all the fun things they have to offer.

After lunch at a locally-owned, hole-in-the-wall café in this town, you amble over to the park near the town center and sit on a park bench, chatting with your significant other (or with the friend who accompanied you on this day), discussing what you both liked (and disliked) about this cute little town that neither of you had ever explored before.

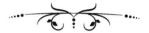

It's August, and you wake up in an unfamiliar bed. You take a quick shower in an unfamiliar shower, then you head downstairs and walk into the kitchen, where your son (or daughter) and their spouse are sitting together, each drinking coffee and reading the newspaper.

They hop up when you walk into the kitchen and offer to cook breakfast for you. Then the three of you pass a pleasant morning chatting as you catch up on all the things that have been going on in their family's life, and you fill them in on all the things that have been going on in your own life.

Eventually, your grandkids come tearing into the kitchen and give you a hug and a kiss. You spend the morning playing with your grandkids, and eventually duck away for a much-needed nap (how did you ever have so much energy in those years gone by when you were raising your own kids?).

You pass the afternoon watching a movie with your grandkids then going on a nice, quiet walk with your son/daughter. After dinner, all of you play a board game together, and then you climb into bed at night with a huge smile on your face.

The smile is partly there because of how rewarding it is to spend time around your grandkids, and to see how well your own child is doing...but that smile is also partly there because you will be going back home tomorrow.

As wonderful as it is to be around your child, your grandchildren, and this family you love so much, you also have so many rewarding things awaiting you in your own life, and you are very much looking forward to getting back to those things.

It's September, and you wake up to a day you cannot exactly say you have been "looking forward to," but nevertheless, you hop out of bed and force a smile onto your face.

No one likes moving, after all...but hey, it's always nice to do something to help others. And anyway, you promised your friend that you would help them when it came time for them to move to their new house, and a promise is a promise.

You made certain to wake up earlier than you needed to on this day in order to be able to start the day on the right foot; having a quiet, relaxing breakfast and getting "centered" (making a concerted, intentional effort to reach a place of complete inner peace), before having to spend the day helping a friend do something you hope to never have to do yourself again.

Much to your surprise, however, the day of moving is not nearly as overwhelming as you had expected it to be. Your friend made sure everything was packed and organized before "moving day" arrived, and they were able to enlist a number of other friends to help with the effort. Each of you does your part, and the day passes fairly quickly and efficiently.

In the afternoon, all of you stop for a big lunch (provided, graciously, by the friend who is moving, and whom all of you are helping). Then, feeling replenished from the food and the break, all of you hit it hard for the remainder of the day, completing the loading of the moving truck, then driving to the new house and helping to unload everything.

When the day ends, you offer to return the next day and help your friend unpack the boxes and start setting up the house...but thankfully, they turn down your offer to help. As you drive home, you reflect on how happy you are that you made the effort to help. After all, even though it may not always be easy, it sure feels nice to contribute to the lives of others.

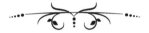

It's October, and the crisp air is knocking the brightly colored leaves off the tree. You watch through the window for a few minutes as these leaves drift toward the ground, then you hop out of bed and take a quick shower and head to the kitchen to put together the sandwiches and the snacks for the picnic you have planned for the day: you and a close friend (or your significant other) are going to load up the bicycles, take a scenic ride through the colorful leaves, then have a picnic in the park.

The two of you take things fairly easy on the bikes, deciding to turn this into a pleasant, leisurely experience, rather than turning it into an intense workout (a decision that is perfectly fine by you), and you pause every now and then to climb off the bikes and walk around areas with particularly pretty colors to the leaves.

After a couple of hours of riding the bikes and enjoying all the beauty around you, the two of you unload the picnic you have prepared, spread a blanket in the grass, and dive in. After you finish eating, you remain sitting on the blanket for a while, enjoying the pleasant ambiance of the perfect autumn day and feeling excessively happy.

Finally, you pack up the items from the picnic, load the now-empty picnic basket onto the back of your bike once more, and ride back to the car, drinking in the twilight of this perfect autumn day.

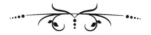

It's November, and although it is certainly not something you would call "fun," it is definitely one of the most rewarding things you do each year. After breakfast, you will be driving downtown to the homeless shelter, where you volunteer each year for the Thanksgiving dinner they provide to the homeless in the area.

You arrive at the homeless shelter early enough to help them with the last hour or so of setup and food preparation, and then the doors open and you take your place behind the table where you will be spooning mashed potatoes onto the plates of those who make their way down the line.

Every year, when you volunteer for this event, you are both surprised and impressed by how pleasant, cordial, and downright grateful the individuals are as they pass through the line.

As the morning bleeds into afternoon, you hit your stride, feeling more comfortable and regularly engaging in conversation with those who make their way down the line. You smile at them and sometimes even offer words of encouragement; they smile in return and thank you for the food and for your kindness.

By the time the afternoon ends and the last of the homeless individuals make their way down the line, you begin to wish there was more you could do to help them. But while you may not have as much money as you would like to have for making the world a better place for those who find themselves in this unfortunate situation, you resolve to look for something you can do each month at the homeless shelter, in order to really contribute to the solution in this sad area of humanity.

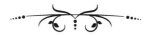

It's December, and Christmas is a couple of weeks away, but, of course, you have long-ago realized that "Christmas" is about more than just Christmas Day itself; instead, Christmas is about the entire season, and you generally attempt to do all you can do enjoy every aspect of this season that is available for you to enjoy.

Because it is a Saturday, you know the mall will be busy, and this is exactly the kind of day you look forward to at this time of year. You have a hard time finding a parking spot (no surprise there), but eventually you find one and make the long walk toward the entrance to the mall.

For a little while, you wander around and watch the shoppers (one of your favorite Christmas traditions these days), and eventually you treat yourself to some food from the food court and find a bench to sit on in the mall. From this bench, you can see the line of children waiting to see Santa Claus; you can see the shoppers bustling by; you can see a number of the brightly-decorated storefronts; and you can hear the Christmas music (most of it far more raucous than the Christmas music you prefer) that they play throughout the mall.

By the time you leave the mall, as much as you enjoy the opportunity to people-watch in such a frenetic and Christmas-driven setting, you are ready for some peace and quiet. You head home and relax for a bit, and then you decide to leave the house at night and drive through a few nearby neighborhoods to enjoy the Christmas lights that are hung on the houses.

You play Christmas music in your car (the kind of soft, pleasant Christmas music you prefer) as you drive slowly through the neighborhoods and take in the festive atmosphere, then you head home and pop in your favorite Christmas movie and watch it for a bit, until you finally get too tired to stay up any longer and you go to bed at last.

HOW TO GET THERE...

You can be an "exceptional retired individual." You simply need to know how to get there...

Look, I know that each of us is unique. Each of us is different. No two of us are alike. I know that it is overwhelmingly unlikely that everything I described in the previous chapter will apply to you as something you see as being part of "the perfect life."

But I also wanted to take you on that journey, to place you inside that journey, because I feel it is important for you to understand just how full and complete retired life can be. There are so many things to do in this world. There are so many ways to enjoy life.

Most people, throughout their working years, can hardly wait to retire so they can finally have the time to enjoy these things at last. And then they retire and they make no effort to enjoy any of these things at all. Perhaps there are days early on in their retired years when they wake up and think about doing some of these things.

It seems easier to simply stay in (just for "that day," of course...naturally, none of these people plan to make "staying in and doing nothing particularly rewarding or valuable" their permanent state of life, but it starts with one day, and another day gets added, and so on... and all the momentum begins to build in the wrong direction).

On the other hand, there are those "exceptional retired individuals" who wake up each day and either have a plan as to how they are going to make this day fulfilling, memorable, and rewarding, or have an openness to the sort of spontaneity that can turn a "normal day" into a day that is instead fulfilling, memorable, and rewarding.

These are the sorts of individuals who come to see life as a great adventure, instead of seeing it as something to just "get through." These are the sorts of individuals who end up "thriving" through their retired years...instead of just "surviving."

Again, I know that not everything in the previous chapter applies to you or illustrates, for you, a "perfect life," but I also feel it is important for you to gain a picture of just how full and rewarding life can be, yes, even for retired individuals. In fact, I will go so far as to say, *especially* for retired individuals.

As such, it will be important for you to also come to understand what it will take for you to reach that "perfect life," a life in which each day *matters* and in which you are truly thriving, instead of simply surviving.

Of course, if you are reading this as someone who is not yet in your 60s, 70s, 80s, or 90s, as someone who is not yet retired, one of the best things you can do (as discussed earlier), is to start leading an exceptional life *now*.

If you can start treating each day as a gift, as something exciting, something worth enjoying, something worth cherishing (yes, even when it is nothing more than a "work day"), you will put yourself in a tremendous position to be able to get more out of your retired years than most people ever come close to getting.

But even if you are retired already, even if you are already in your 60s, 70s, 80s, or 90s, and you did not build this habit during your working years, there are things you can do to "get there." There are things you can do to live life as an "exceptional retired individual."

There are things you can do to help you reach a place where you are LIVING LONGER AND BETTER, getting the most out of life and genuinely *thriving*, instead of living a life in which you are simply "surviving."

It all starts with your outlook. When you think of yourself, how do you see yourself? Do you see yourself as "old"? Do you see your life as being "limited"? Do you think that all your best years are behind you, and that there is really not a whole lot left for you besides, you know, just trying to not get too sick? If any of these sound like you, it's time to wake up.

Each of us wants to lead a life that is fulfilling, rewarding, and worthwhile, but most of us never pause to consider the fact that such a life does not simply come our way by accident. In order to have a life that fulfills those criteria, you need to approach life in a manner that is conducive to fulfilling those criteria, and this will ultimately mean having a positive outlook, one that leads you toward positive and rewarding activity in your life.

The sooner you stop seeing yourself as "old," and the sooner you stop picturing your life as something that is largely "limited," the sooner you will be able to start living a life that is truly worth living.

It's worth repeating: *A fulfilling, rewarding, worthwhile life does not come your way by accident.* Instead, you need to be *intentional* about making your life as fulfilling, rewarding, and worthwhile as you want it to be, and the first step in this process will be acknowledging that there is still plenty of life ahead of you, and that there are plenty of reasons why it is still worth your time and effort to make the most of each and every day. When you can reach this point, you will find that you are on the right path to leading that "perfect life" at last.

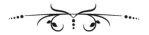

A large portion of this book, of course, deals with the intangible areas of your life that you need to take care of in order to *LIVE LONGER AND BETTER*, your mental acuity, your emotional well-being, and your spiritual depth, as well as the things you should be proposing to do in your life in order to actually make each day worth living.

The things you should be doing in order to create enjoyable, rewarding experiences in your life that will ensure you are "thriving" each day instead of "just surviving." And the reason I have placed such a heavy focus on these sides of this topic is because these are the contributing elements to LIVING LONGER AND BETTER that are talked about the least.

After all, you can do all you want in the way of health, wellness, and fitness, and can still end up experiencing that unwanted, early deterioration in both your mind and your body if you are failing to take the proper steps toward enhancing your mental, emotional, and spiritual well-being.

But as true as this is, the reverse of it is true as well. If you are taking great care of your mental, emotional, and spiritual well-being, this will certainly be great for your ability to LIVE LONGER AND BETTER, but none of this will mean anything if you are failing to take proper care of your body.

Now, naturally, there are hundreds (possibly even thousands) of books available that deal with all the specific things you can be doing in order to take care of your physical fitness and your body as a senior, which is why I have chosen to focus more heavily on those areas of *LIVING LONGER AND BETTER* that are talked about far less frequently; your mental, emotional, and spiritual well-being.

But even with the importance of those elements toward ensuring you are A) living a long, healthy life, and B) enjoying life to the fullest for as long as you are around, you need to realize that this all stacks up to nothing if you are failing to take care of your body. Because of this, you need to start looking for the things you can do to keep yourself active, each and every day.

Yes. I said, "Each and every day."

Every day, you should be eating healthily. That's a given. And every day, you should be making sure you are getting a healthy amount of sleep. But also, every day, you should be engaging in some form of physical activity that will contribute to your body's long-term health, fitness, and well-being.

Of course, this does not necessarily need to be something strenuous every day, but you have to do more walking than just making your way from the bedroom to the living room, or from the living room to the kitchen.

Maybe, for you, it's walking. Maybe it's water aerobics or simply swimming laps in the pool. Maybe it's bike riding, or maybe it's weightlifting. Maybe it's a dance class or yoga. Maybe it's a mixture of those things. Maybe it's all of the above, or maybe it is something that is not even on that list.

Regardless of what it is, you need to find something you can do that will keep you active and will help to ensure your body is in the best position possible for remaining strong and healthy. And then, you need to make the effort to engage in these activities every single day.

If you are having a difficult time achieving the level of physical activity you should be achieving in order to ensure the long-term health and fitness of your body, a great way to turn the tide is by setting goals. What do you want to work toward physically? What are you hoping to accomplish?

One of the greatest benefits of "setting goals" is that it helps to direct your physical activity in a specific manner, toward a specific end. For example, for years, I have enjoyed working out, but when I decided to begin doing triathlons, I found that my workouts were now more focused and specifically-tailored, as these workouts were largely dedicated toward reaching a level of specific physical fitness that would enable me to compete in the triathlons in which I aimed to compete.

Of course, now that I am in triathlon shape, I am able to also focus on other areas of strength and fitness, but I had to first follow a specific path in order to be physically prepared to accomplish a specific goal.

In the chapter detailing "the perfect life," one of the examples we took you through was a hike up a mountain. If you chose, right now, to hike up a mountain, is this something you would be able to do? For most of us, the answer to that question would be "No." So let's say, then, that you had a group of friends with whom you wanted to attempt to climb a mountain.

If this were the case, you would then have a specific goal toward which you were moving in your workouts, and would be able to tailor your workouts and your daily "physical fitness efforts" toward ensuring you would be prepared to climb that mountain by the date you had set.

Then, once you have reached that place of physical fitness and have climbed that mountain, you will be able to set a new goal, and this new goal can once more direct your workouts.

In the chapter in which I detailed the things you can/should be doing for your body, for your mind, for your emotions, and for your spirituality, the last point listed for each was that you should be "intentional." You probably noticed this yourself...and this means you probably do not need me to tell you that "living intentionally" is a huge, huge deal.

One of the best ways to "live intentionally" is by taking the time to actually stop and think about what you want to see in your life in each of the areas discussed in this book (your body, your mind, your emotions, and your spirituality). By thinking about what you want to see in each of these areas, and by then writing down what you would like to see in each of these areas, you will put yourself in a position from which you can actively work toward reaching these goals and bringing these ideas to fruition in your own life.

What's more, I like to encourage people to write down their idea of a "perfect life." What is your idea of a "perfect life"? (Is this something you have ever even thought about before?)

Is your idea of a "perfect life" waking up, rolling out of bed, and watching television until it is time to go to bed again? Or does your idea of a "perfect life" encompass more than this? Stop to think about it; really ponder this question, and then, write down what you see as the fulfillment of the "perfect life," and figure out the ways in which you should be "living intentionally," each and every day, to make this "perfect life" your own reality.

How is your mental state?

How is your emotional state?

How is your spirituality?

In addition to setting goals for health and physical fitness in order to be able to strive toward these goals, and in addition to knowing what your "perfect life" looks like (and writing this down in order to be able to actively work toward making this "perfect life" the life you are living yourself), you should also write down the things you can be doing (the things you should be doing) each and every day to enhance your mental state, your emotional state, and your spirituality.

This, of course, ties into "living intentionally," but it also serves the all-important focus of giving you some specific direction in your efforts to "live intentionally" toward a desired end.

The more *intentional* you are with your body, your mind, your emotions, and your spirituality, the better position you will be in to effectively *LIVE LONGER AND BETTER*.

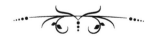

After you have come up with a list of the things you can (should) be doing each and every day in order to A) get the most out of life, and B) continually enhance the state of your body, mind, emotions, and spirituality, it will also be extraordinarily beneficial for you to keep a log of what your days look like. Yes, each and every day.

Now, for some, this can take the form of a journal or a diary, in which you not only jot down what that day looked like, but in which you also take a bit of time to express your thoughts and (on a continuous, day-to-day manner) assess your life.

Of course, this can help quite a bit in ensuring that you are actually improving each day and are constantly moving toward a "perfect life," as most of us do not really verbalize our thoughts or self-evaluations until we make a concerted effort to do so.

By taking the time at the end of each day to write down our uninhibited thoughts, and our honest opinions on how the day went (and of how we handled our own self that day in our quest to *LIVE LONGER AND BETTER*, our quest to "thrive," rather than just to "survive"), we will have a sort of built-in, daily evaluation tool that will put us in the best possible position for continually improving and continually brightening our future.

While it is certainly great to take this approach; keeping a daily journal or diary can have a tremendously positive impact on our ability to truly move into the full, fulfilled life we desire to live, I also understand that not all of us are inclined to keep a journal or a diary.

Not all of us can take the time to do this each and every day (or even if we can take the time, many of us will, if being completely honest with ourselves, admit that this is something we *will* not actually take the time to do each day, even if we have the best intentions of doing so).

But even if this is not something you can (or will) do, you can replicate a lot of the benefits of a daily journal/diary by simply keeping a daily log. What did your day look like? What did you do that day? What fulfilling, rewarding, memorable activity or situation defined your day?

When you know that the end of each day will include an entry in your daily log, an entry in which you must account for your day and quantify its impact on both your present (*LIVING BETTER*) and your future (*LIVING LONGER*), you will find that you are automatically becoming far more "intentional" with each and every day.

After all, do you really want to open your daily log and have to write down, "Today, I did nothing truly worthwhile"? Do you want to write down, "Today, I did nothing that significantly improved my body, my mind, my emotions, or my spirituality"?

Or do you instead want to be able to open your daily log, pick up your pen, and write down some brief notes about all the awesome, rewarding, memorable things your day contained.

Once again, keeping a true journal or diary, in which you take a bit of time each day to genuinely spill your thoughts and have a self-assessment, is (by far) one of the best ways to ensure you are living intentionally and are continually improving your life every single day.

But even if you do not take the 15 or 20 minutes required each day in order to do that, you should, at the very least, keep a daily log in which you close out each day by briefly jotting down what your day looked like, and in which you note the ways in which you truly enjoyed the present and built toward your future.

With this "accountability system" built into each and every day of your life, it will become far more difficult for you to be sloppy with the approach you are taking to each day, and it will significantly increase the chances of you making the most of each day that comes your way.

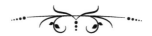

It may sound simple, but once you have the knowledge of what it means to *LIVE BETTER*, and of what it takes to *LIVE LONGER*, all that truly remains is for you to be intentional; in the steps you are taking to make the idea of *LIVING LONGER AND BETTER* a reality in your own life, of the steps you are taking, that is to say, to ensure that you are "thriving," instead of simply "surviving." And the best way to put yourself in the position to live *intentionally* is this: Assess, improve, and enjoy each day...then repeat.

When you assess each day, you will make yourself consciously aware of the steps you are taking in order to truly live and enjoy the "perfect life" for you. And when you take your assessment and then determine the ways in which you would like to improve the next day, you will ensure that each day is set up to be better than the day before, thereby creating a life comprised of a string of constantly-improving days.

And finally, you will need to make sure you are always "living in the moment," enjoying each day for the gift that it is, instead of spending each day thinking about the future, or thinking about your past, or thinking about all those "hectic thoughts" (trying to corral and gather all those bouncing balls of "little things that do not really even matter").

Assess, improve, and enjoy each day...then repeat.

When you are able to reach a place where your life looks like this, you will truly be in a position to fully enjoy the gift of each day, and will be constantly *LIVING BETTER,* while always building toward *LIVING LONGER.*

Live intentionally.

Assess, improve, and enjoy each day...then repeat.

That's what *LIVING LONGER AND BETTER* is really all about.

LIVING BETTER: A RECAP

It's time to stop "surviving"; it is time, instead, to start thriving.

Each and every one of us has a different idea of exactly what "the perfect life" looks like. This is, of course, quite natural, as each of us has our own dreams, desires, likes, and dislikes, our own ideas of what it means to "live better," and our own ideas of what it means to "thrive." But even through all this, there is one thing that just about every single one of us can agree on:

It is better to lead a healthy, happy life than to lead a life that is neither healthy nor happy.

And this is what the idea of *LIVING LONGER AND BETTER*, the idea of thriving instead of surviving, is really all about.

Each of us has the ability to lead a life that not only stretches into our 90s (or even into our 100s), but, more importantly, each of us has the ability to lead a life that stretches deep into these years, while also ensuring that this life continues to be healthy and rewarding. Each of us can lead a fulfilled life that lasts far longer than what most people imagine.

Each of us can make the most of this time we have on Earth, all while stretching this time out far longer than most people realize it can be stretched. And now that you have read this book, you also have the tools and the knowledge necessary to start down this path yourself.

Of course, leading a healthy lifestyle is a big part of *LIVING LONGER AND BETTER*. You need to make an effort to remain active, you need to eat healthy, you need to get enough sleep, and you need to stay away from overmedication. You need to take care of your physical body in order to give yourself the best chance possible of leading a truly long and rewarding life.

But while this is the area that is talked about the most, and is the area most people (and most doctors) will tend to focus on, it is not going to be enough, on its own, to ensure that you are in the best possible

LIVING BETTER: A RECAP

position to lead a long, healthy, fulfilling life. In addition to taking care of yourself physically, you need to keep your mind sharp, engaged, and healthy.

After all, your brain is the command center for your entire body. With a sharp, healthy mind, you will not only put your body itself in a better position to carry you to many healthy years, but you will also ensure that your mind is in a position to help you actually enjoy these years. What good is it to have a healthy body, but to have a mind that is not sharp enough to ensure you are able to enjoy the present?

And of course, in addition to taking care of your body and your mind, you need to also place a strong focus on your emotional health and stability. Emotional health has a much greater impact on physical and mental health than most people ever take the time to realize, and if you are not actively managing your emotions, you are not going to ever be able to experience the fullness of life that is available to you.

And finally, you need to pay attention to your spirituality. You need to connect with something greater than yourself, and you need to push yourself to a place from which you are able to experience a high level of inner peace, reaching a place where you feel "centered" and stable at all times, as this will have a huge impact on your emotional health, your mental health, and your physical health.

Yes, it may be a bit of work to *LIVE LONGER AND BETTER*. It may require you to take a bit of an active interest in all areas of your health and life if you are going to truly enjoy a long, fulfilling life. But it is truly worth it. And yes, it truly does matter...

WHY DOES IT MATTER?

"Does it really matter if I am able to live longer and better?" Yes, it absolutely does.

As a society, we like to ask questions. We like to challenge things we have heard. We like to push the limits and break free from what we see as the "status quo." We hear things others have said, and we want to search out these things on our own, never taking the words of others at face value, but instead digging deeper, seeing what we are able to uncover beneath the surface.

This is often a good thing. It is this type of thinking, after all, that ultimately pushes a society forward. It is this type of thinking that enables us to come up with new ideas and that enables us to uncover truths through which our lives are made better.

It is also this kind of thinking, however, that can cause us to question even the most obvious truths. It is this kind of thinking that can lead someone to read a book such as this and to ask, "Yes, but why does it matter?" Why does it matter if we, as a society, learn to *LIVE LONGER AND BETTER*?

While we could probably fill an entire book with the reasons why it is better for the people in our society to *LIVE LONGER AND BETTER*, we are going to save that lengthy discussion for another time. For now, instead, we are going to take a brief look at the core reasons why it is better for individuals themselves, for the families of these individuals, and for the world as a whole if we can all start learning to *LIVE LONGER AND BETTER*.

The Individual

Every once in a while, you will hear someone say something like this: "I don't really want to live beyond the age of 75 or so." When you ask this person why they feel this way, however, their explanation will almost always stretch into the fact that they do not want to be old and sick; instead, they want to lead a full life, and then they would prefer to die before things start going downhill too rapidly.

But what would these people say if they were presented with an alternative? What if they were assured that they would be able to live until, say, 95 years of age (instead of 75 years of age), and would be able to enjoy tremendous health and a fulfilling day-to-day life all the way to that age? Would they still say that they would prefer to simply leave this world at the age of 75, or would they instead agree that they would prefer to have those extra 20 years of fulfilled living available to them?

You see? The overwhelming majority of people who are not interested in *LIVING LONGER* feel this way because they equate the idea of "living longer" with the idea of sickness, turmoil, and a difficult decline. There are very few individuals, however, who would say that the idea of both "living longer" AND "living better" fails to appeal to them. Life, after all, when lived to the fullest, is a tremendous gift.

Regardless of the age you are right now, as you read this book, you probably agree that you would love to live longer if you were enjoying a healthy, fulfilled life all those years you were alive. Do you agree? Do you feel that you would prefer to have more years available to you, assuming you are able to use those years to enjoy the beauty in the world, to enjoy friends, to enjoy family, to enjoy the gift of life?

Would you prefer to live longer if you could have fun with those extra years, if you could use those years to really and truly *LIVE* life...to really and truly "thrive," instead of simply "surviving"?

Quite simply, this is why it matters to the individual to be able to *LIVE LONGER AND BETTER*. Sure, "living longer" may not sound like the most appealing idea in the world if your idea of "living longer" goes hand-in-hand with thoughts of deteriorating mental health, physical health, and lifestyle; or if your idea of "living longer" also coincides with a concept of "requiring more help from others" and "leading a handicapped and fully-assisted life"; but if you are able to *LIVE LONGER* while also *LIVING BETTER*, most people would agree that there is really no reason why they would not want to stick around for as many years as possible.

The Individual's Family

"Burden."

This is, sadly, one of the words most often ascribed to an older individual in a family. This older individuals who should be called a treasure, who should be viewed as a source of wisdom and knowledge, who should be respected and held in high regard, and who should be looked up to and adored, is often said to be a "burden."

This older individual in the family who is largely responsible for not only the existence of those who have come after them, but who is also responsible for much of the knowledge and learning, much of the "leg up in life" many of the younger individuals in the family have been blessed with, ends up being seen as nothing more than a drain on time and money.

It sounds sad, doesn't it? It sounds completely wrong. But at the same time, for those who are in the younger generation and are tasked with looking after the older members of the family, who must spend their money to take care of the older members of the family, and must invest large chunks of time to "making life easy on" this rapidly-declining individual, it is often difficult to truly view this older individual as the treasure they are.

After all, we as humans are, for the most part, fundamentally concerned with ourselves first and foremost, and this is not necessarily a bad thing in fact, as it is difficult to take care of someone else if we are not first taking care of ourselves. And because of this fundamental disposition toward self-care and self-preservation, it can become quite natural to have a hard time mentally and emotionally when much of our "own time" (time during which we would like to firstly be taking care of ourselves and secondly be taking care of the family members we are supposed to be primarily taking care of, our spouse, and our children) is dedicated, instead, to taking care of an adult who took care of their own self for so long.

Is it right for younger people to feel this way when tasked with taking care of an older family member? Of course not. But is it natural for them to feel this way? Quite honestly, it absolutely is.

For all the joy and pleasure available in life, life is, in many ways, challenging. It's not always easy to find the time to build our life into what we want it to be. And it is not always easy to build up the money we need to build up in order to have an optimal life before us.

When an individual's time and money suddenly must start going toward "easing the transition" of an older family member, it can place a strain on not only that individual's present, but on their future as well. Money that was saved for that individual's children goes, instead, toward their parents (or grandparents, or aunts and uncles).

Time that should be dedicated toward building up the strength of that individual's family and improving the future prospects of their own children is instead poured into monitoring the rapid decline of that "older family member." This makes it difficult for the individual in question taking care of that older family member with a good attitude, sure, but more importantly, it also puts that individual in a bind as they move forward into their own future.

This becomes a self-perpetuating cycle. The individual who is pouring time and money into taking care of their older family members is now at a disadvantage themselves, in their own efforts to ensure their children will not have to do the same for them. And so, years later, they become that "older family member," and their children must now take care of them and "ease their transition." The cycle continues.

When, on the other hand, these "older family members" are able to continue "thriving" deep into their years, the burden on the younger family members is made far lighter. What's more, these older family members are able to pour more time, effort, energy, and wisdom into the younger family members (children, grandchildren, great-grandchildren, etc.), which leads to the rest of the family being made stronger and becoming even more prepared to thrive themselves, in their own lives.

As older family members *LIVE LONGER AND BETTER*, they end up contributing to the ability of others in their family, younger members of their family, to do the same in their own lives.

This is a self-perpetuating cycle that any family would want to see take place. This is a cycle that benefits all involved. This is a cycle that makes the future of an entire family far brighter than it would otherwise be.

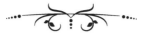

Society

How much money is spent each year in Medicaid and Medicare? Do you have a guess? Hundreds of thousands of dollars? Millions of dollars? *Billions* of dollars?

Try this: Roughly $1 trillion dollars are spent every year in Medicaid and Medicare. That is money spent every single year in order to help the older members of our society, and more often than not, this money is not spent helping people who are LIVING LONGER AND BETTER, but is instead spent taking care of people in decline...helping to ease the decline for these individuals, and helping to make life "less uncomfortable" as they "survive" for a few more years.

Will there be spending required for the care and treatment of older individuals in our country, no matter how fully we are able to grasp this idea of LIVING LONGER AND BETTER? Of course there will be.

If we, as a society, can begin this revolution toward no longer "surviving," but toward instead "thriving" deep into our years on Earth, the financial burden "older individuals" have on each country will rapidly decrease. Instead of being seen as a "burden," these individuals will begin to be seen for what they truly are; a blessing to our society, and to the wisdom, learning, and knowledge of younger generations.

Yes, it is time for us, as a society, to learn what we can do to start *LIVING LONGER AND BETTER.* It is time to start the revolution, to change the way we see those post-retirement years, and to move into the bright, new future that lays in wait before us.

YOUR JOURNEY STARTS NOW

It is time, today, right this very moment, in fact, to take the first steps. It is time to start your journey toward LIVING LONGER AND BETTER.

It does not matter who you are. It does not matter what age you are, or what your past looks like, or where you are in your present. It does not matter what your family's medical history is or even what your personal medical history is. It does not matter what you have believed up until now. The fact still stands: It is entirely possible for you to start *LIVING LONGER AND BETTER.*

You can lead a fulfilled life.

You can "thrive," instead of simply "surviving."

You can be an "exceptional retired individual."

You can break the mold and fight the status quo and truly enjoy all that life has to offer.

Yes, you can *LIVE LONGER*. You can *LIVE BETTER*.

You can enjoy the sort of physical, mental, emotional, and spiritual health that most people only dream of enjoying late into life. You can lead the way to a new way of retired living.

Are you ready?

Your journey starts today...

Your journey starts now.

About
Dr. Andrew Scanameo

Dr. Scanameo is an anti-aging specialist with a dedicated private practice in geriatric medicine in Tallahassee Florida.

He is a New York native who did his training at Rutgers-UMDNJ medical campus in New Jersey and went on to complete his geriatric training at Mount Sinai Hospital in Manhattan.

He holds board certifications in Internal Medicine, Geriatrics and Hospice/Palliative care medicine.

He has extensive research experience and his published works include The Molecular Basis of Dementia as well as guides to visiting patients at home. He has won multiple awards including a national Award for his work in the biochemical basis of Alzheimer's Disease.

He has dedicated his professional life and his personal life to longevity. His devotion to health and fitness is witnessed by the fact that he is an active triathlete and enjoys participating in races in North Florida.

For More Information Visit Dr. Andrew's Website at:

www.ElderParentCentral.com

Made in the USA
Columbia, SC
16 April 2019